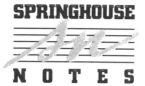

SPRINGHOUSE

N O T E S

MEDICAL SURGICAL NURSING

Mildred W. Boyd, RN, MSN

Ms. Boyd, a coauthor of this book, is an Assistant Professor of Nursing at Essex Community College, Baltimore County, Md. She earned her BSN from the University of Maryland at College Park and received her MSN from Boston University. Ms. Boyd is a member of Alpha Eta and is listed in *Who's Who in American Nursing*.

Barbara L. Tower, RN, MA, MSN, CCRN

Ms. Tower, a coauthor of this book, is an Assistant Professor of Nursing at Essex Community College, Baltimore County, Md. She earned her BA and MA from Florida State University, Tallahassee, her BSN from the State University of New York at Plattsburgh, and her MSN from the Catholic University of America, Washington, D.C. Ms. Tower is a member of Sigma Theta Tau and the American Association of Critical-Care Nurses and is a Mellon Fellow.

Sr. Esther D. Holzbauer, MSN

Sr. Holzbauer, the reviewer of this book, is an Assistant Professor of Nursing at Mount Marty College, Yankton, S.D. She earned her BSN from Mount Marty College and received her MSN from the University of Nebraska at Omaha.

Springhouse Publishing Company
Springhouse, Pennsylvania

STAFF FOR THIS VOLUME

CLINICAL STAFF

Clinical Director
Barbara McVan, RN

Clinical Editors
Lynne Atkinson, RN, BSN, CEN
Joan E. Mason, RN, EdM
Diane Schweisguth, RN, BSN, CCRN, CEN

ADVISORY BOARD

Mildred Wernet, Boyd, RN, BSN, MSN
Assistant Professor, Essex Community College, Baltimore

Dorothy Brooten, PhD, FAAN
Chairperson, Health Care of Women and Childbearing Section, Director of Graduate Perinatal Nursing, University of Pennsylvania School of Nursing, Philadelphia

Lillian S. Brunner, MSN, ScD, LittD, FAAN
Nurse/Author, Brunner Associates, Inc., Berwyn, Pa.

Irma J. D'Antionio, RN, PhD
Professor, Parent-Child Nursing, University of Pittsburgh, School of Nursing, Pittsburgh

Kathleen Dracup, RN, DNSc, FAAN
Associate Professor, School of Nursing, University of California, Los Angeles

Cecile A. Lengacher, RN, PhD
Director of the Division of Nursing and Health Sciences, Manatee Junior College, Bradenton, Fla.

Barbara Tower, RN, MSN, CCRN
Assistant Professor, Essex Community College, Baltimore

PUBLICATION STAFF

Executive Director, Editorial
Stanley Loeb

Executive Director, Creative Services
Jean Robinson

Design
John Hubbard (art director), Stephanie Peters (associate art director), Jacalyn Bove Facciolo, Julie Carleton Barlow

Editing
Donna L. Hilton (acquisitions), Kathy E. Goldberg, Patricia McKeown, David Prout

Copy Editing
David Moreau (manager), Edith McMahon (supervisor), Nick Anastasio, Keith de Pinho, Diane Labus, Doris Weinstock, Debra Young

Art Production
Robert Perry (manager), Anna Brindisi, Christopher Buckley, Loretta Caruso, Donald Knauss, Christina McKinley, Mark Marcin, Robert Wieder

Typography
David Kosten (manager), Diane Paluba (assistant manager), Joyce Rossi Biletz, Alicia Dempsey, Brenda Mayer, Nancy Wirs

Manufacturing
Deborah Meiris (manager), Lisa Weiss

Project Coordination
Aline S. Miller (supervisor), Maureen Carmichael

The clinical procedures described and recommended in this publication are based on research and consultation with nursing, medical, and legal authorities. To the best of our knowledge, these procedures reflect currently accepted practice; nevertheless, they can't be considered absolute and universal recommendations. For individual application, all recommendations must be considered in light of the patient's clinical condition and, before administration of new or infrequently used drugs, in light of latest package-insert information. The authors and the publisher disclaim responsibility for any adverse effects resulting directly or indirectly from the suggested procedures, from any undetected errors, or from the reader's misunderstanding of the text.

© 1988 by Springhouse Corporation, 1111 Bethlehem Pike, Springhouse, Pa. 19477. All rights reserved. Reproduction in whole or part by any means whatsoever without written permission of the publisher is prohibited by law. Authorization to photocopy items for internal or personal use, or the internal or personal use of specific clients, is granted by Springhouse Corporation for users registered with the Copyright Clearance Center (CCC) Transactional Reporting Service, provided that the base fee of $00.00 per copy plus $.75 per page is paid directly to CCC, 27 Congress St., Salem, MA 01970. For those organizations that have been granted a photocopy license by CCC, a separate system of payment has been arranged. The fee code for users of the Transactional Reporting Service is: 0874341132/88 $00.00 + $.75.

Printed in the United States of America.

SN7-061290

Library of Congress Cataloging-in-Publication Data

Boyd, Mildred W.
   Medical-surgical nursing/Mildred W. Boyd, Barbara L. Tower; [reviewed by] Esther D. Holzbauer.
   p. cm.—(Springhouse notes)
   Includes bibliographies and index.
   ISBN 0-87434-113-2
   1. Nursing.   2. Surgical nursing.   I. Tower, Barbara L.   II. Holzbauer, Esther D.   III. Title.
   IV. Series.
   [DNLM: 1. Nursing Care.   2. Surgical nursing.
   WY 150 B789m]
   RT41.B64   1988   610.73—dc19
   DNLM/DLC
   for Library of Congress   87-26707
                                                          CIP

Contents

How to Use Springhouse Notes

Today, more than ever, nursing students face enormous time pressures. Nursing education has become more sophisticated, increasing the difficulties students have with studying efficiently and keeping pace.

The need for a comprehensive, well-designed series of study aids is great, which is why we've produced Springhouse Notes...to meet that need. Springhouse Notes provide essential course material in outline form, enabling the nursing student to study more effectively, improve understanding, achieve higher test scores, and get better grades.

Key features appear throughout each book, making the information more accessible and easier to remember.
- **Learning Objectives.** These objectives precede each section in the book to help the student evaluate knowledge before and after study.
- **Key Points.** Highlighted in color throughout the book, these points provide a way to quickly review critical information. Key points may include:
—a cardinal sign or symptom of a disorder
—the most current or popular theory about a topic
—a distinguishing characteristic of a disorder
—the most important step of a process
—a critical assessment component
—a crucial nursing intervention
—the most widely used or successful therapy or treatment.
- **Points to Remember.** This information, found at the end of each section, summarizes the section in capsule form.
- **Glossary.** Difficult, frequently used, or sometimes misunderstood terms are defined for the student at the end of each section.

Remember: Springhouse Notes are learning tools designed to *help* you. They are not intended for use as a primary information source. They should never substitute for class attendance, text reading, or classroom note taking.

This book, *Medical-Surgical Nursing,* is organized by body system. The sections, each covering one body system, include the following information: anatomy and physiology, physical assessment findings, diagnostic tests and procedures, possible psychosocial impact, possible risk factors, actual and potential nursing diagnoses, surgical interventions, and medical disorders. Each surgical intervention covers all pertinent information necessary to provide preoperative and postoperative nursing care. Each medical disorder includes information necessary to provide nursing care, including pathophysiology and a reference list of possible surgical interventions. Medical and nursing interventions may include more than one option in the progression of care and must be prioritized and adapted to meet individual patient needs. Keep in mind that many nursing interventions, such as medications, require a doctor's order.

Cardiovascular System

Learning Objectives

After studying this section, the reader should be able to:

- Describe the psychosocial impact of cardiovascular system disorders.

- Differentiate between modifiable and nonmodifiable risk factors in the development of a cardiovascular system disorder.

- List three potential and three actual nursing diagnoses for the patient with a cardiovascular system disorder.

- Identify the medical and surgical nursing interventions/responsibilities for patients with a cardiovascular system disorder.

- Write three teaching goals for the patient with a cardiovascular system disorder.

I. Cardiovascular System

A. Anatomy and physiology
1. Heart
   a. Muscular organ: composed of two atria and two ventricles surrounded by pericardial sac
   b. Two-layered pericardial sac: visceral (inner) and parietal (outer)
   c. Three-layered heart wall: epicardium (visceral pericardium), myocardium, endocardium
   d. Four valves: tricuspid, mitral, pulmonic, aortic
   e. Myocardial blood supply: left (LCA) and right (RCA) coronary arteries; LCA branches into left anterior descending (LAD) and circumflex arteries; collateral circulation
   f. Electrical conduction: impulse initiated by sinoatrial (SA) node ("intrinsic pacemaker"), atrial depolarization, atrial contraction (P wave), atrioventricular (AV) node, bundle of His, left and right bundle branches, Purkinje fibers, ventricular depolarization, ventricular contraction (QRS complex), ventricular repolarization (T wave)
   g. Blood flow: blood returns to heart from inferior and superior vena cava to right atrium, through tricuspid valve to right ventricle, through pulmonic valve to pulmonary artery, to lungs, to pulmonary veins to left atrium, through mitral valve to left ventricle, through aortic valve to aorta and systemic circulation
   h. Cardiac function: cardiac output (CO) is total amount of blood ejected per minute; stroke volume (SV) is amount of blood ejected with each beat; $CO = SV \times HR$ (heart rate)
2. Blood vessels
   a. Arteries are three-layered vessels (intima, media, adventitia) that carry oxygenated blood from the heart to the tissues
   b. Arterioles are small resistance vessels that feed into capillaries
   c. Capillaries join arterioles to venules, which are where nutrients and wastes are exchanged
   d. Venules are larger, lower-pressured vessels than arterioles and join capillaries to veins
   e. Veins are large capacity, low-pressure vessels that return unoxygenated blood to the heart

B. Physical assessment findings
1. Subjective data that often accompany cardiovascular disorders
   a. Dyspnea
   b. Paroxysmal nocturnal dyspnea (PND)
   c. Orthopnea
   d. Chest and leg pain
   e. Fatigue and weakness
   f. Cough
   g. Syncope
   h. Palpitations

2. Objective data to evaluate in cardiovascular disorders
    a. Blood pressure
    b. Pulses
    c. Skin color and temperature
    d. Heart sounds
    e. Edema
    f. Dysrhythmias
    g. Jugular venous distention (JVD)
    h. Respiratory distress
    i. Vascular bruits
    j. Location of point of maximum impulse (PMI)
    k. Jaundice
    l. Pruritus

C. **Diagnostic tests and procedures used to evaluate cardiovascular disorders**
    1. Electrocardiography (EKG)
        a. Definition/purpose: noninvasive test that graphically represents the electrical activity of the heart
        b. Nursing interventions/responsibilities: assess ability of patient to lie still; reassure patient that electrical shock will not occur
    2. Ambulatory electrocardiography (Holter monitoring)
        a. Definition/purpose: noninvasive recording of the electrical activity of the heart over 24 hours
        b. Nursing interventions/responsibilities: instruct patient to record activity diary; instruct patient not to bathe or shower, operate machinery, or use microwave ovens or electric shavers
    3. Cardiac catheterization
        a. Definition/purpose: fluoroscopic examination of intracardiac structures, pressures, oxygenation, and CO after injection of a radiopaque dye
        b. Nursing interventions/responsibilities: before procedure, withhold food and fluids after midnight; obtain baseline vital signs (VS) and peripheral pulses; obtain written, informed consent; instruct patient that he may experience nausea, chest pain, flushing of the face, or throat irritation when dye is injected; assess allergies to seafood, iodine, or radiopaque dyes; after procedure, monitor VS, peripheral pulses, and injection site for bleeding; maintain pressure dressing and bed rest; force fluids unless contraindicated; allay anxiety
    4. Echocardiography
        a. Definition/purpose: noninvasive examination that uses echoes from sound waves to visualize intracardiac structures and direction of blood flow
        b. Nursing interventions/responsibilities: assess patient's ability to lie still; explain the procedure
    5. Exercise testing (stress)
        a. Definition/purpose: noninvasive study of electrical activity of the heart during prescribed levels of exercise

   b. Nursing interventions/responsibilities: withhold food and fluids 1 hour
      before test; instruct patient to wear loose-fitting clothing and supportive
      shoes; explain the procedure
6. Nuclear cardiology
   a. Definition/purpose: visual imaging of myocardial perfusion and
      contractility after I.V. injection of radioisotopes
   b. Nursing interventions/responsibilities: explain the procedure; allay
      anxiety; assess patient's ability to lie still during the procedure
7. Coronary arteriography
   a. Definition/purpose: fluoroscopic examination of coronary arteries after
      injection of a radiopaque dye
   b. Nursing interventions/responsibilities: before procedure, assess allergies
      to iodine, seafood, or radiopaque dyes; monitor VS; allay anxiety;
      inform patient he may feel flushing of the face or throat irritation after
      dye is injected; after procedure, assess insertion site for bleeding; assess
      peripheral pulses; maintain pressure dressing and bed rest
8. Digital subtraction angiography
   a. Definition/purpose: invasive procedure using computer system and
      fluoroscopy with image intensifier to permit complete visualization of
      arterial supply to specific area
   b. Nursing interventions/responsibilities: before procedure, obtain written,
      informed consent; monitor VS; after procedure, assess insertion site for
      bleeding, instruct patient to drink at least 1 liter of fluid
9. Hemodynamic monitoring
   a. Definition/purpose: examination of intracardiac pressures and CO using a
      balloon-tipped, flow-directed catheter (Swan-Ganz)
   b. Nursing interventions/responsibilities: before procedure, obtain written,
      informed consent; after procedure, assess insertion site for signs of
      infection; monitor pressure tracings; record readings
10. Chest X-ray
   a. Definition/purpose: radiographic picture of the heart and lungs
   b. Nursing interventions/responsibilities: assess patient's ability to hold his
      breath; remove jewelry
11. Blood chemistries
   a. Definition/purpose: laboratory analysis of blood sample for sodium,
      potassium, magnesium, calcium, glucose, phosphorus, cholesterol,
      triglycerides, uric acid, bicarbonate, creatinine (Cr), blood urea nitrogen
      (BUN), bilirubin, creatinine phosphokinase (CPK), CPK isoenzymes,
      lactic dehydrogenase (LDH), LDH isoenzymes, serum glutamic
      oxaloacetic transaminase (SGOT)
   b. Nursing interventions/responsibilities: assess site for bleeding; withhold
      food and fluids as ordered; note drugs that may interfere with test;
      restrict exercise before blood sample is drawn; hold intramuscular
      injections or note time of injection on laboratory slip

12. Hematologic studies
    a. Definition/purpose: laboratory analysis of blood sample for red blood cells (RBC), white blood cells (WBC), erythrocyte sedimentation rate (ESR), prothrombin time (PT), partial thromboplastin time (PTT), platelets, hemoglobin (Hgb), and hematocrit (Hct)
    b. Nursing interventions/responsibilities: assess site for bleeding; note drugs that may interfere with test
13. Arterial blood gases (ABGs)
    a. Definition/purpose: assessment of arterial blood for tissue oxygenation, ventilation, and acid-base status
    b. Nursing interventions/responsibilities: document temperature, supplemental oxygen, and assisted mechanical ventilation used before testing; after procedure, assess site for bleeding and maintain pressure dressing
14. Doppler ultrasound
    a. Definition/purpose: noninvasive examination that uses echoes from sound waves that are then transformed into audible sounds to assess the blood flow in the peripheral circulation
    b. Nursing interventions/responsibilities: assess the patient's ability to lie still; explain the procedure
15. Venogram
    a. Definition/purpose: visualization of the veins after I.V. injection of a dye to diagnose deep vein thrombosis or incompetent valves
    b. Nursing interventions/responsibilities: before procedure, withhold food and fluids after midnight; obtain baseline VS and peripheral pulses; obtain written, informed consent; assess allergies to seafood, iodine, or radiopaque dyes; inform patient he might feel flushing of face or burning in the throat after dye is injected; after procedure, assess injection site for bleeding and hematoma, force fluids unless contraindicated

D. **Possible psychosocial impact of cardiovascular disorders**
    1. Developmental impact
        a. Fear of rejection
        b. Decreased self-esteem
        c. Fear of dying
        d. Role conflict
    2. Economic impact
        a. Disruption or loss of employment
        b. Cost of hospitalization
        c. Cost of special diets
        d. Cost of medications
    3. Occupational and recreational impact
        a. Restrictions in work activity
        b. Change in leisure activity

    c. Restrictions in physical activity (stairs, walking)

    d. Restrictions in activity related to environmental temperature

  4. Social impact

    a. Change in dietary habits

    b. Change in sexual function

    c. Change in role performance

    d. Social isolation

E. **Possible risk factors for the development of cardiovascular disorders**

  1. Modifiable risk factors

    a. Smoking

    b. Hypertension

    c. Hypercholesterolemia

    d. Obesity

    e. Physical inactivity

    f. Emotional stress

  2. Nonmodifiable risk factors

    a. Gender

    b. Family history of cardiovascular illness

    c. Childhood history of cardiovascular illness

    d. Ethnic background

    e. Racial background

    f. Aging process

F. **Possible nursing diagnoses for the patient with a cardiovascular disorder**

  1. Actual nursing diagnoses

    a. Alteration in cardiac output: decreased

    b. Alteration in comfort: pain

    c. Alteration in tissue perfusion: cardiopulmonary

    d. Alteration in tissue perfusion: peripheral

    e. Alteration in tissue perfusion: cerebral

  2. Potential nursing diagnoses

    a. Alteration in fluid volume: excess

    b. Activity intolerance

    c. Fear

    d. Anxiety

    e. Ineffective individual coping

    f. Ineffective family coping: compromised

    g. Disturbance in self-concept: self-esteem

    h. Disturbance in self-concept: role performance

    i. Disturbance in self-concept: body image

    j. Sexual dysfunction

    k. Noncompliance

G. Surgical intervention: cardiac surgery
1. Definition
    a. Coronary artery bypass graft (CABG): surgical revascularization of the coronary arteries using saphenous veins or internal mammary artery to bypass an obstruction caused by atherosclerosis
    b. Valve replacement: surgical replacement of stenotic or incompetent valves with a mechanical or bioprosthetic valve such as Starr-Edwards "ball-in-cage" valves, porcine valves, Bjork-Shiley "tilting disk" valves
    c. Valvular annuloplasty: surgical repair or reconstruction of the leaflets and annulus of the valve
    d. Mitral valve commissurotomy: surgical opening of the fused portion of the mitral valve leaflets using a dilator
    e. Valvuloplasty: surgical repair or reconstruction of the valve
2. Preoperative surgical nursing interventions/responsibilities
    a. Complete patient and family preoperative teaching: assess understanding of surgical procedure; explain operating room (OR), recovery room (RR), preoperative, and postoperative routine; demonstrate postoperative turning, coughing, and deep-breathing (TCDB), splinting, leg exercises and range-of-motion (ROM) exercises; explain postoperative need for drainage tubes, surgical dressings, oxygen therapy, I.V. therapy, and pain control
    b. Allay patient and family anxiety about surgery
    c. Document patient history and physical assessment data base
    d. Obtain baseline hemodynamic variables, EKG, and ABGs
    e. Complete preoperative check list
    f. Administer preoperative medications
3. Postoperative surgical nursing interventions/responsibilities
    a. Assess cardiac, respiratory, neurologic status, and fluid balance
    b. Assess pain and administer postoperative analgesic
    c. Progress diet as tolerated after extubation
    d. Administer I.V. fluids and transfusion therapy
    e. Allay anxiety
    f. Assess surgical dressing and change as directed
    g. Reinforce TCDB and splinting of incision
    h. Maintain semi-Fowler position
    i. Assess for return of peristalsis
    j. Provide pulmonary toilet: incentive spirometry after extubation, endotracheal suction
    k. Maintain activity: as tolerated, active and passive ROM, isometric exercises
    l. Administer oxygen and maintain endotracheal tube to ventilator
    m. Monitor VS, urine output (UO), intake/output (I/O), laboratory studies, EKG, hemodynamic variables, daily weights
    n. Monitor and maintain position and patency of drainage tubes: nasogastric (NG), Foley, wound drainage, chest

      o. Encourage ventilation of feelings about change in body image, fear of dying

      p. Administer antibiotics

      q. Monitor, record, and maintain chest drainage system to water seal for mediastinal and pleural chest tubes

      r. Monitor dysrhythmias

      s. Assess peripheral circulation: color, temperature, pulses, sensation

      t. Administer antiarrhythmics

      u. Administer anticoagulants

      v. Administer vasopressors

      w. Administer beta adrenergics

      x. Administer diuretics

      y. Administer cardiac glycosides

      z. Have temporary pacemaker available

4. Possible surgical complications

      a. Bleeding from mediastinal tube

      b. Perioperative MI

      c. Decreased cardiac output

      d. Dysrhythmias

      e. Cardiac tamponade

      f. Heart block

      g. Embolism

      h. Valve malfunction

5. Patient/family postoperative teaching goals; the patient will:

      a. Keep follow-up appointments

      b. Maintain regular exercise program

      c. Stop smoking

      d. Maintain ideal weight

      e. State the action, side effects, and scheduling of medications

      f. Recognize the signs and symptoms of infection and bleeding

      g. Avoid driving and heavy lifting for 6 weeks

      h. Complete daily incision care

      i. Elevate saphenous graft site leg when seated

      j. Wear antiembolitic stockings

      k. Maintain low-sodium diet

H. Surgical intervention: abdominal aneurysm resection

1. Definition: surgical removal of a portion of weakened arterial wall with an end-to-end anastomosis to a prosthetic graft

2. Preoperative surgical nursing interventions/responsibilities

      a. Complete patient and family preoperative teaching: assess understanding of surgical procedure; explain OR, RR, preoperative, and postoperative routine; demonstrate postoperative TCDB, splinting, leg exercises, and ROM; explain postoperative need for drainage tubes, surgical dressings, oxygen therapy, I.V. therapy, and pain control

      b. Complete preoperative check list

     c. Administer preoperative medications

     d. Allay patient and family anxiety about surgery

     e. Document patient history and physical assessment data base

3. Postoperative surgical nursing interventions/responsibilities (as ordered)

     a. Assess cardiac, respiratory, neurologic status, and fluid balance

     b. Assess pain and administer postoperative analgesic

     c. Progress diet as tolerated

     d. Administer I.V. fluids and transfusion therapy

     e. Allay anxiety

     f. Assess surgical dressing and change as directed

     g. Reinforce TCDB and splinting of incision

     h. Maintain flat position with turning side to side

     i. Assess for return of peristalsis

     j. Provide pulmonary toilet: incentive spirometry after extubation, endotracheal suction

     k. Maintain activity: bedrest, active and passive ROM, isometric exercises

     l. Administer oxygen and maintain endotracheal tube to ventilator

     m. Monitor VS, UO, I/O, central venous pressure (CVP), laboratory studies, EKG, hemodynamic variables

     n. Monitor and maintain position and patency of drainage tubes: NG, Foley

     o. Measure abdominal girth

     p. Assess peripheral circulation: color, temperature, sensation, pulses in extremities

     q. Assess for scrotal and retroperitoneal bleeding

     r. Administer antibiotics

4. Possible surgical complications

     a. Renal failure

     b. Atelectasis

     c. Graft hemorrhage

5. Patient/family postoperative teaching goals; the patient will:

     a. Keep follow-up appointments

     b. Maintain regular exercise program

     c. Stop smoking

     d. Maintain ideal weight

     e. State the action, side effects, and scheduling of medications

     f. Recognize the signs and symptoms of infection

     g. Avoid lifting, bending, and driving

     h. Complete daily incision care

     i. Monitor blood pressure daily

     j. Identify and reduce stress

     k. Adhere to low-sodium, low-cholesterol diet

I. Surgical intervention: vascular grafting

1. Definition

     a. Surgical revascularization of an artery, using a synthetic or autogenous graft to "bypass" or resect the diseased segment

   b. Types: femoropopliteal, aortofemoral, aortoiliac, femorofemoral, axillofemoral
2. Preoperative surgical nursing interventions/responsibilities
   a. Complete patient and family preoperative teaching: assess understanding of surgical procedure; explain OR, RR, preoperative, and postoperative routine; demonstrate postoperative TCDB, splinting, leg exercises, and ROM; explain postoperative need for drainage tubes, surgical dressings, oxygen therapy, I.V. therapy, and pain control
   b. Complete preoperative check list
   c. Administer preoperative medications
   d. Allay patient and family anxiety about surgery
   e. Document patient history and physical assessment data base
   f. Obtain baseline assessment of peripheral circulation
   g. Administer antibiotics
3. Postoperative surgical nursing interventions/responsibilities
   a. Assess cardiac and neurovascular status
   b. Assess pain and administer postoperative analgesic
   c. Progress diet as tolerated
   d. Administer I.V. fluids and transfusion therapy
   e. Allay anxiety
   f. Assess surgical dressing and change as directed
   g. Reinforce TCDB and splinting of incision
   h. Maintain semi-Fowler position; avoid positioning and flexion on graft site
   i. Assess for return of peristalsis
   j. Provide pulmonary toilet: incentive spirometry
   k. Maintain activity: as tolerated, active and passive ROM, isometric exercises
   l. Monitor VS, UO, I/O, laboratory studies, neurovascular checks
   m. Monitor and maintain position and patency of drainage tubes: NG, Foley
   n. Encourage ventilation of feelings about change in body image
   o. Measure abdominal girth
   p. Assess peripheral circulation: temperature, color, pulses, and sensation in extremities distal to graft site
   q. Measure ankle, calf, and thigh circumference
   r. Progress ambulation
   s. Provide bed cradle
   t. Administer anticoagulants
4. Possible surgical complications
   a. Thrombosis
   b. Embolus
   c. Graft rejection
   d. Hemorrhage
5. Patient/family postoperative teaching goals; the patient will:
   a. Keep follow-up appointments
   b. Maintain regular exercise program
   c. Stop smoking
   d. Maintain ideal weight

  e. State the action, side effects, and scheduling of medications
  f. Recognize the signs and symptoms of infection of the graft site
  g. Avoid positions that put pressure on or flex the graft site
  h. Avoid wearing constrictive clothing
  i. Complete daily incision care
  j. Protect graft site from injury
  k. Check pulses distal to graft site daily
  l. Adhere to long-term anticoagulant therapy
  m. Wear properly fitting shoes
  n. Maintain daily foot care

J. Hypertension
  1. Definition: constant elevation of systolic or diastolic blood pressure (greater than 140/90 mm Hg)
  2. Possible etiology
      a. Unknown etiology for primary hypertension
      b. Renal disease
      c. Pheochromocytoma
      d. Cushing's disease
  3. Pathophysiology
      a. Diameter of the arterioles is narrowed, resulting in increased peripheral resistance
      b. Increased peripheral resistance requires increased force to circulate blood, resulting in increased blood pressure
  4. Possible clinical manifestations
      a. Asymptomatic
      b. Elevated blood pressure
      c. Headache
      d. Visual disturbances
      e. Left ventricular hypertrophy
      f. Renal failure
      g. Dizziness
      h. Papilledema
      i. CHF
      j. Cerebral ischemia
  5. Possible diagnostic test findings
      a. Blood pressure: sustained reading greater than 160/95 mm Hg
      b. EKG: Left ventricular hypertrophy
      c. Chest X-ray (CXR): Cardiomegaly
      d. Ophthalmoscopic examination: retinal changes
      e. Blood chemistry: increased sodium, cholesterol
  6. Medical management
      a. Diet therapy: low-sodium, low-calorie, low-cholesterol
      b. I.V. therapy: heparin lock
      c. Activity: ad lib
      d. Monitoring: VS, UO, EKG, I/O

    e. Laboratory studies: sodium, potassium, cholesterol
    f. Diuretics: furosemide (Lasix), spironolactone (Aldactone), hydrochlorothiazide (Hydrodiuril)
    g. Antihypertensives: methyldopa (Aldomet), hydralazine (Apresoline), prazosin (Minipress)
    h. Vasodilators: sodium nitroprusside (Nipride)
    i. Calcium blockers: nifedipine (Procardia), verapamil (Calan), diltiazem (Cardizem)
    j. Beta-adrenergic blockers: propranolol (Inderal), metoprolol (Lopressor)

7. Medical nursing interventions/responsibilities
    a. Maintain diet
    b. Assess cardiovascular status
    c. Monitor and record VS, UO, I/O, laboratory studies, daily weights
    d. Administer medications
    e. Encourage ventilation of feelings about daily stressors
    f. Provide a quiet environment

8. Patient/family teaching goals; the patient will:
    a. Keep follow-up appointments
    b. Maintain regular exercise program
    c. Stop smoking
    d. Maintain ideal weight
    e. State the action, side effects, and scheduling of medications
    f. Identify and reduce stress
    g. Follow dietary restrictions and recommendations
    h. Maintain quiet environment

9. Possible medical complications
    a. Cerebrovascular accident (CVA)
    b. Visual changes
    c. Renal failure
    d. CHF
    e. Hypertensive crisis

10. Possible surgical interventions: none

K. Coronary artery disease: arterio/atherosclerosis

1. Definition
    a. Arteriosclerosis: "hardening of the arteries," which results in loss of elasticity of intimal layer of the artery
    b. Atherosclerosis: accumulation in the arteries of fatty plaques made of lipids

2. Possible etiology
    a. Aging process
    b. Stress
    c. Genetics
    d. Depletion of estrogen

3. Pathophysiology
   a. Coronary arteries are narrowed or obstructed by the accumulation of plaque, the presence of an embolus, or vasospasm
   b. The narrowing or obstruction of the artery results in decreased perfusion and inadequate myocardial oxygen supply
4. Possible clinical manifestations
   a. Angina
   b. MI
   c. CHF
   d. Sudden death
   e. Hypertension
5. Possible diagnostic test findings
   a. EKG: ST depression, T wave inversion
   b. Stress test: abnormal EKG, chest pain
   c. Coronary arteriography: plaque formation
   d. Blood chemistry: increased cholesterol
   e. Ambulatory electrocardiography: ST depression, T wave inversion
6. Medical management
   a. Diet therapy: low-calorie, low-sodium, low-cholesterol
   b. I.V. therapy: heparin lock
   c. Oxygen therapy
   d. Monitoring: VS, UO, CVP, EKG, hemodynamic variables, I/O, neurovascular checks
   e. Laboratory studies: sodium potassium, cholesterol, CPK, LDH, SGOT, CPK isoenzymes, LDH isoenzymes, ABGs
   f. Weight reduction
   g. Arterial line for blood pressure (BP) monitoring
   h. Intraaortic balloon pump (IABP)
   i. Streptokinase therapy
   j. Percutaneous transluminal coronary angioplasty (PTCA)
   k. Treatments: Foley catheter
   l. Antihyperlipidemic agents: cholestyramine (Questran), clofibrate (Atromid-S)
   m. Nitrates: nitroglycerin, isosorbide dinitrate (Isordil)
   n. Beta-adrenergic blockers: propranolol (Inderal), nadolol (Corgard)
   o. Calcium blockers: nifedipine (Procardia), verapamil (Calan), diltiazem (Cardizem)
   p. Analgesics: morphine (MS Contin)
   q. Antianxiety agents: diazepam (Valium)
7. Medical nursing interventions/responsibilities
   a. Maintain diet
   b. Administer oxygen
   c. Assess cardiovascular status
   d. Monitor and record VS, UO, hemodynamic variables, I/O, EKG, laboratory studies

    e. Administer medications
    f. Encourage ventilation of feelings about fear, anxiety
  8. Patient/family teaching goals; the patient will:
    a. Keep follow-up appointments
    b. Maintain regular exercise program
    c. Stop smoking
    d. Maintain ideal weight
    e. State the action, side effects, and scheduling of medications
    f. Identify and reduce stress
    g. Differentiate between the pain of angina and the pain of myocardial infarction
    h. Adhere to activity limitations
    i. Limit alcohol intake to 2 ounces per day
    j. Monitor blood pressure daily
    k. Follow dietary restrictions and recommendations
  9. Possible medical complications
    a. Angina
    b. MI
    c. CHF
  10. Possible surgical interventions: CABG (see page 11)

L. Angina
  1. Definition: chest pain from inadequate myocardial oxygen supply
  2. Possible etiology
    a. Atherosclerosis
    b. Vasospasm
    c. Aortic stenosis
    d. Activities or disease that increase metabolic demands
  3. Pathophysiology
    a. Narrowing of coronary arteries results from plaque accumulation in intimal lining of artery
    b. Plaque accumulation obstructs blood flow, which diminishes myocardial oxygen supply
  4. Possible clinical manifestations
    a. Pain: substernal, crushing, compressing pain, which may radiate to arms, lasting 3 to 5 minutes after exertion, exposure to cold, or emotional excitement
    b. Dyspnea
    c. Palpitations
    d. Epigastric distress
    e. Tachycardia
    f. Patient history: chest pain with activity
    g. Diaphoresis
    h. Anxiety
    i. Pain at rest

5. Possible diagnostic test findings
   a. EKG: ST depression, T wave inversion during an acute episode of pain
   b. Stress test: abnormal EKG, chest pain
   c. Coronary arteriography: plaque accumulation
   d. Blood chemistry: increased cholesterol
   e. Cardiac enzymes: within normal limits
   f. Ambulatory electrocardiography: ST depression, T wave inversion
6. Medical management
   a. Diet therapy: low-calorie, low-sodium, low-cholesterol
   b. I.V. therapy: heparin lock
   c. Oxygen therapy
   d. Position: semi-Fowler
   e. Monitoring: VS, UO, EKG, hemodynamic variables, I/O, neurovascular checks
   f. Laboratory studies: ABGs, sodium, potassium, CPK with isoenzymes, LDH with isoenzymes, SGOT
   g. PTCA
   h. Streptokinase therapy
   i. Arterial line for blood pressure monitoring
   j. Nitrates: nitroglycerin (Nitro-Bid), isosorbide dinitrate (Isordil)
   k. Beta-adrenergic blockers: propranolol (Inderal), nadolol (Corgard)
   l. Calcium blockers: verapamil (Calan), diltiazem (Cardizem), nifedipine (Procadia)
7. Medical nursing interventions/responsibilities
   a. Maintain diet
   b. Administer oxygen
   c. Assess cardiovascular status
   d. Monitor and record VS, UO, hemodynamic variables, I/O, laboratory studies, chest pain
   e. Administer medications
   f. Encourage ventilation of feelings about fear, anxiety
   g. Encourage rest at onset of pain
   h. Take EKG during an acute attack
   i. Maintain semi-Fowler position
8. Patient/family teaching goals; the patient will:
   a. Keep follow-up appointments
   b. Maintain regular exercise program
   c. Stop smoking
   d. Maintain ideal weight
   e. State the action, side effects, and scheduling of medications
   f. Identify and reduce stress
   g. Differentiate between the pain of angina and the pain of myocardial infarction
   h. Avoid activities that result in angina: exertion, heavy meals, exposure to cold environment, emotional upsets

      i. Alternate rest periods with activity
      j. Follow dietary restrictions and recommendations
      k. Seek medical attention if pain lasts more than 20 minutes
      l. Monitor blood pressure daily

9. Possible medical complications
    a. Dysrhythmias
    b. CHF
    c. MI

10. Possible surgical interventions: CABG (see page 11)

M. Myocardial infarction (MI)

1. Definition: death of portion of myocardial muscle cells related to lack of oxygen from inadequate perfusion
2. Possible etiology
    a. Atherosclerosis
    b. Decreased perfusion
    c. Embolism or thrombus
    d. Coronary artery spasm
3. Pathophysiology
    a. Coronary arteries are narrowed with plaque accumulation that causes critical reduction in perfusion and death of myocardial cells secondary to lack of oxygen
    b. Myocardial cells die due to inadequate perfusion and oxygenation from a complete obstruction of the vessel
4. Possible clinical manifestations
    a. Substernal crushing pain that may radiate to jaw, back, and arms; lasts longer than anginal pain; unrelieved by rest or nitroglycerin; may be asymptomatic ("silent MI")
    b. Dyspnea
    c. Nausea and vomiting
    d. Anxiety
    e. Diaphoresis
    f. Pallor
    g. Dysrhythmias
    h. Increased temperature
5. Possible diagnostic test findings
    a. EKG changes: enlarged Q wave, elevated ST segment, T wave inversion
    b. Blood chemistry: increased CPK, LDH, SGOT, lipids; positive CPK-MB fraction, flipped LDH-1 and LDH-2 isoenzymes
    c. Hematology: increased WBC
6. Medical management
    a. Diet therapy: low-calorie, low-cholesterol, low-fat
    b. Antiarrhythmics: quinidine (Quinaglute), lidocaine (Xylocaine), procainamide (Pronestyl)
    c. Anticoagulants: aspirin (Ecotrin)
    d. Antihypertensives: hydralazine (Apresoline), methyldopa (Aldomet)

      e. IABP

      f. Left ventricular assist device (LVAD)

      g. Streptokinase therapy

      h. Monitoring: VS, UO, EKG, hemodynamic variables

      i. Oxygen therapy

      j. Laboratory studies: ABGs, CPK, CPK isoenzymes, LDH, LDH isoenzymes, SGOT, WBC, sodium, potassium, glucose

      k. Position: semi-Fowler

      l. I.V. therapy: heparin lock

      m. PTCA

      n. Arterial line for blood pressure monitoring

7. Medical nursing interventions/responsibilities

      a. Maintain diet

      b. Assess cardiovascular and respiratory status

      c. Monitor and record VS, UO, I/O, hemodynamic variables, laboratory studies, EKG

      d. Maintain bed rest

      e. Administer oxygen therapy

      f. Administer medications

      g. Take EKG during an acute episode of pain

      h. Allay anxiety

      i. Maintain semi-Fowler position

      j. Provide rest periods

8. Patient/family teaching goals; the patient will:

      a. Keep follow-up appointments

      b. List the action, side effects, and scheduling of medications

      c. Identify and reduce stress

      d. Maintain regular exercise program

      e. Stop smoking

      f. Demonstrate a change in life-style

      g. Follow dietary recommendations and restrictions

      h. Participate in cardiac rehabilitation program

      i. Maintain ideal weight

      j. Differentiate between the pain of angina and the pain of myocardial infarction

      k. Alternate rest periods with activity

9. Possible medical complications

      a. Dysrhythmias

      b. Cardiogenic shock

      c. CHF

      d. Papillary muscle rupture

      e. Pericarditis

      f. Sudden cardiac death

10. Possible surgical interventions: CABG (see page 11)

N. Congestive heart failure: left-sided
1. Definition: failure of the left side of the heart to pump enough blood to meet the metabolic demands of the body
2. Possible etiology
    a. Atherosclerosis
    b. Fluid overload
    c. MI
    d. Valvular stenosis
    e. Valvular insufficiency
    f. Hypertension
    g. Cardiac conduction defects
3. Pathophysiology
    a. Decreased myocardial contractility or increased myocardial workload results in increased left ventricular pressure, increased left atrial pressure, and decreased CO
    b. Increased pressure in the pulmonary capillaries leads to decreased oxygenation and respiratory manifestations of fluid overload
4. Possible clinical manifestations
    a. Dyspnea
    b. PND
    c. Rales
    d. Cough
    e. Gallop rhythm: S3, S4
    f. Dysrhythmias
    g. Fatigue
    h. Anxiety
    i. Orthopnea
    j. Tachycardia
    k. Tachypnea
5. Possible diagnostic test findings
    a. CXR: increased pulmonary congestion, left ventricular hypertrophy
    b. Echocardiography: increased size of chambers and decreased wall motion
    c. Hemodynamic monitoring: increased pulmonary capillary wedge pressure (PCWP), CVP, pulmonary artery (PA) pressure, decreased CO
    d. ABGs: hypoxemia, hypercapnea
    e. EKG: left ventricular hypertrophy
    f. Blood chemistry: decreased potassium, sodium; increased BUN, Cr
6. Medical management
    a. Diet therapy: low-sodium; restrict fluids
    b. I.V. therapy: electrolyte replacement; heparin lock
    c. Oxygen therapy
    d. Position: semi-Fowler
    e. Activity: bed rest, active ROM, isometric exercises
    f. Monitoring: VS, UO, I/O, EKG, hemodynamic variables
    g. Laboratory studies: ABGs, sodium, potassium, BUN, Cr
    h. Treatments: Foley catheter

    i. IABP
    j. LVAD
    k. Analgesics: morphine sulfate (Roxanol)
    l. Diuretics: furosemide (Lasix), ethacrynic acid (Edecrin)
    m. Vasodilators: sodium nitroprusside (Nipride)
    n. Cardiac inotropes: dopamine HCl (Intropin), dobutamine (Dobutrex)
    o. Cardiac glycosides: digoxin (Lanoxin)
    p. Nitrates: isosorbide dinitrate (Isordil), nitroglycerin (Nitro-Bid)
7. Medical nursing interventions/responsibilities
    a. Maintain diet
    b. Restrict fluids
    c. Administer I.V. fluids
    d. Administer oxygen
    e. Provide pulmonary toilet: suction, TCDB
    f. Assess cardiovascular and respiratory status
    g. Weigh daily
    h. Maintain semi-Fowler position
    i. Monitor and record VS, UO, CVP, hemodynamic variables, I/O, laboratory studies
    j. Assess peripheral edema
    k. Administer medications
    l. Encourage ventilation of feelings about fear of dying
8. Patient/family teaching goals; the patient will:
    a. Keep follow-up appointments
    b. Stop smoking
    c. Maintain ideal weight
    d. State the action, side effects, and scheduling of medications
    e. Supplement diet with foods high in potassium and low in sodium
    f. Recognize signs and symptoms of fluid overload
    g. Adhere to activity limitations
    h. Alternate rest periods with activity
    i. Follow dietary recommendations and restrictions
9. Possible medical complications
    a. Digitalis toxicity
    b. Fluid overload
    c. Cardiogenic shock
    d. Pulmonary edema
    e. Hypokalemia
10. Possible surgical interventions: none

O. Congestive heart failure: right-sided
1. Definition: failure of the right side of the heart to pump enough blood to meet the metabolic demands of the body
2. Possible etiology
    a. Atherosclerosis
    b. Left-sided CHF

    c. Chronic obstructive pulmonary disease (COPD)

    d. Valvular stenosis

    e. Valvular insufficiency

3. Pathophysiology

    a. Pressure increases from left-sided failure continue to progress with "backward failure"

    b. Venous congestion increases in the systemic circulation with fluid overload

4. Possible clinical manifestations

    a. JVD

    b. Anorexia

    c. Nausea

    d. Ascites

    e. Hepatomegaly

    f. Dependent edema

    g. Weight gain

    h. Signs of left-sided failure

    i. Gallop rhythm: S3, S4

    j. Tachycardia

    k. Fatigue

5. Possible diagnostic test findings

    a. CXR: pulmonary congestion, cardiomegaly, pleural effusions

    b. Echocardiogram: increased size of chambers, decrease in wall motion

    c. Hemodynamic monitoring: increased PCWP, PA pressure, CVP; decreased CO

    d. ABGs: hypoxemia

    e. EKG: left and right ventricular hypertrophy

    f. Blood chemistry: decreased sodium, potassium; increased BUN, Cr

6. Medical management

    a. Diet therapy: low-sodium; restricted fluids

    b. I.V. therapy: electrolyte replacement, heparin lock

    c. Oxygen therapy

    d. Position: semi-Fowler

    e. Activity: bed rest, active ROM, isometric exercises

    f. Monitoring: VS, UO, I/O, EKG, hemodynamic variables

    g. Laboratory studies: ABGs, sodium, potassium, BUN, Cr

    h. Treatments: Foley catheter

    i. IABP

    j. Thoracentesis

    k. Paracentesis

    l. Analgesics: morphine sulfate (Roxanol)

    m. Diuretics: furosemide (Lasix), ethacrynic acid (Edecrin)

    n. Vasodilators: sodium nitroprusside (Nipride)

    o. Cardiac inotropes: dopamine HCl (Intropin), dobutamine (Dobutrex)

    p. Cardiac glycosides: digoxin (Lanoxin)

    q. Nitrates: isosorbide dinitrate (Isordil), nitroglycerin (Nitro-Bid)

7. Medical nursing interventions/responsibilities
   a. Maintain diet
   b. Restrict fluids
   c. Administer I.V. fluids
   d. Administer oxygen
   e. Provide pulmonary toilet: suction, TCDB
   f. Assess cardiovascular and respiratory status
   g. Assess peripheral edema
   h. Maintain semi-Fowler position
   i. Monitor and record VS, UO, I/O, hemodynamic variables, laboratory studies
   j. Weigh daily
   k. Administer medications
   l. Encourage ventilation of feelings about fear of death
   m. Measure abdominal girth
8. Patient/family teaching goals; the patient will:
   a. Keep follow-up appointments
   b. Weigh daily
   c. Stop smoking
   d. Maintain ideal weight
   e. State the action, side effects, and scheduling of medications
   f. Supplement diet with foods high in potassium and low in sodium
   g. Recognize signs and symptoms of fluid overload
   h. Adhere to activity limitations
   i. Alternate rest periods with activity
   j. Follow dietary recommendations and restrictions
9. Possible medical complications
   a. Digitalis toxicity
   b. Fluid overload
   c. Cardiogenic shock
   d. Pulmonary edema
   e. Hypokalemia
   f. Hypernatremia
10. Possible surgical interventions: none

P. **Acute pulmonary edema**
   1. Definition: most extreme form of left-sided heart failure; results in increased pressure in the capillaries of the lungs and acute transudation of fluid
   2. Possible etiology
      a. Atherosclerosis
      b. MI
      c. Myocarditis
      d. Valvular disease
      e. Smoke inhalation
      f. Drug overdose: heroin, barbiturates, morphine sulfate
      g. Overload of I.V. fluids

3. Pathophysiology
   a. Alveolar and interstitial edema results from failure of the heart to pump adequately
   b. Alveolar and interstitial edema interferes with oxygenation and results in hypoxia
4. Possible clinical manifestations
   a. Dyspnea
   b. Paroxysmal cough
   c. Blood-tinged, frothy sputum
   d. Orthopnea
   e. Tachypnea
   f. Agitation
   g. Restlessness
   h. Intense fear
   i. Chest pain
   j. Syncope
   k. Tachycardia
   l. Cold, clammy skin
   m. Gallop rhythm: S3, S4
   n. JVD
5. Possible diagnostic test findings
   a. CXR: interstitial edema
   b. ABGs: respiratory alkalosis or acidosis
   c. EKG: tachycardia, ventricular enlargement
   d. Hemodynamic monitoring: increased PCWP, CVP, PA pressure; decreased CO
6. Medical management
   a. Diet therapy: low-sodium, restrict fluids
   b. I.V. therapy: electrolyte replacement, heparin lock
   c. Oxygen therapy
   d. Intubation and mechanical ventilation
   e. Rotating tourniquets
   f. Position: semi-Fowler
   g. Activity: bed rest, active ROM, isometric exercises
   h. Monitoring: VS, UO, I/O, EKG, hemodynamic variables
   i. Laboratory studies: sodium, potassium, ABGs, BUN, Cr
   j. Treatments: Foley catheter, endotracheal tube suctioning
   k. Analgesics: morphine sulfate (Roxanol)
   l. Diuretics: furosemide (Lasix), ethacrynic acid (Edecrin)
   m. Vasodilators: sodium nitroprusside (Nipride)
   n. Cardiac inotropes: dopamine HCl (Intropin), dobutamine (Dobutrex)
   o. Cardiac glycosides: digoxin (Lanoxin)
   p. Nitrates: isosorbide dinitrate (Isordil), nitroglycerin (Nitro-Bid)
   q. Bronchodilators: aminophylline (Somophyllin)

7. Medical nursing interventions/responsibilities
   a. Withhold food and fluids
   b. Restrict fluids
   c. Administer I.V. fluids
   d. Administer oxygen
   e. Provide pulmonary toilet: suction, TCDB
   f. Assess cardiovascular and respiratory status
   g. Maintain high-Fowler position
   h. Monitor and record VS, UO, I/O, hemodynamic variables, laboratory studies, daily weights
   i. Allay anxiety
   j. Administer medications
   k. Encourage ventilation of feelings about fear of suffocation
   l. Note color, amount, and consistency of sputum
   m. Apply rotating tourniquets
8. Patient/family teaching goals; the patient will:
   a. Stop smoking
   b. Maintain ideal weight
   c. State the action, side effects, and scheduling of medications
   d. Recognize signs and symptoms of respiratory distress
   e. State signs of fluid overload
   f. Adhere to activity limitations
   g. Alternate rest periods with activity
   h. Follow dietary recommendations and restrictions
   i. Sleep with head of bed elevated
   j. Supplement diet with foods high in potassium and low in sodium
   k. Identify and reduce stress
9. Possible medical complications
   a. Digitalis toxicity
   b. Fluid overload
   c. Pulmonary emboli
   d. Hypokalemia
   e. Hypernatremia
10. Possible surgical interventions: none

Q. Cardiogenic shock
1. Definition: "pump failure" or "power failure" that results in decreased cardiac output and inadequate tissue perfusion
2. Possible etiology
   a. MI
   b. Myocarditis
   c. Advanced heart block
   d. CHF
3. Pathophysiology
   a. The heart fails to pump effectively, resulting in decreased SV and CO and increased left ventricular volume

      b. Compensatory factors of increased HR and increased contractility increase the demand for myocardial oxygen

      c. The imbalance between myocardial oxygen supply and myocardial oxygen demand increases myocardial ischemia, which further compromises the heart's pumping action

4. Possible clinical manifestations
    a. Hypotension: less than 90 mm Hg systolic
    b. Oliguria: less than 30 cc/hour
    c. Cold, clammy skin
    d. Tachycardia
    e. Restlessness
    f. Hypoxia
    g. Tachypnea
    h. Anxiety
    i. Dysrhythmias
    j. Disorientation and confusion

5. Possible diagnostic test findings
    a. ABGs: metabolic acidosis, hypoxemia
    b. EKG: MI (enlarged Q wave, ST elevation)
    c. Blood chemistry: increased BUN, Cr
    d. Hemodynamic monitoring: decreased SV, CO; increased PCWP, CVP, PA pressure

6. Medical management
    a. Diet therapy: withhold food and fluids; restrict fluids
    b. I.V. therapy: electrolyte replacement, heparin lock
    c. Oxygen therapy
    d. Intubation and mechanical ventilation
    e. Position: semi-Fowler
    f. Activity: bed rest, passive ROM, isometric exercises
    g. Monitoring: VS, UO, I/O, EKG, hemodynamic variables, level of consciousness
    h. Laboratory studies: potassium, sodium, BUN, Cr, ABGs
    i. Treatments: Foley catheter, endotracheal tube suction
    j. Circulatory assist devices: IABP
    k. Diuretics: furosemide (Lasix), ethacrynic acid (Edecrin)
    l. Vasodilators: sodium nitroprusside (Nipride)
    m. Cardiac inotropes: dopamine HCl (Intropin), dobutamine (Dobutrex)
    n. Cardiac glycosides: digoxin (Lanoxin)
    o. Vasopressors: norepinephrine (Levophed)

7. Medical nursing interventions/responsibilities
    a. Withhold food and fluids
    b. Limit fluids
    c. Administer I.V. fluids
    d. Administer oxygen
    e. Provide pulmonary toilet: suction, TCDB
    f. Assess cardiovascular and respiratory status, fluid balance

      g. Maintain semi-Fowler position
      h. Monitor and record VS, UO, I/O, hemodynamic variables, level of consciousness, laboratory studies
      i. Administer medications
      j. Encourage ventilation of feelings about fear of death
      k. Allay anxiety
  8. Patient/family teaching goals: the patient will:
      a. Keep follow-up appointments
      b. Maintain regular exercise program
      c. Stop smoking
      d. Maintain ideal weight
      e. State the action, side effects, and scheduling of medications
      f. Identify and reduce stress
      g. Recognize the signs and symptoms of fluid overload
      h. Adhere to activity limitations
      i. Alternate rest periods with activity
      j. Follow dietary recommendations and restrictions
  9. Possible medical complications
      a. Dysrhythmias
      b. Cardiac arrest
      c. Infection
10. Possible surgical interventions: CABG (see page 11)

R. Mitral stenosis
  1. Definition: narrowing of the mitral valve opening
  2. Possible etiology: rheumatic endocarditis
  3. Pathophysiology
      a. Valvular tissue thickens and calcifies, thus narrowing the opening and limiting blood flow from the left atrium to the left ventricle
      b. Limitation of blood flow results in increased pressure in the left atrium, pulmonary hypertension, and left atrial hypertrophy
      c. Right ventricular failure follows, with increased pulmonary congestion and increased workload of the right ventricle
  4. Possible clinical manifestations
      a. Fatigue
      b. Low cardiac output
      c. Dyspnea on exertion
      d. Right-sided heart failure
      e. Cough
      f. Peripheral edema
      g. Atrial fibrillation
      h. Orthopnea
      i. JVD
      j. Tachycardia
      k. PND
      l. Hemoptysis

5. Possible diagnostic test findings
   a. CXR: enlargement of left atrium and right ventricle, pulmonary congestion
   b. Echocardiogram: thickening of mitral valve and left atrial enlargement
   c. Cardiac catheterization: increased left atrial pressure, PCWP; decreased CO
   d. Angiography: mitral stenosis
6. Medical management
   a. Diet therapy: low-sodium, restrict fluids
   b. I.V. therapy: heparin lock
   c. Oxygen therapy
   d. Position: semi-Fowler
   e. Activity: bed rest, active ROM, isometric exercises
   f. Monitoring: VS, UO, I/O, EKG, hemodynamic variables
   g. Laboratory studies: sodium, potassium, PT, PTT, ABGs
   h. Treatments: Foley catheter
   i. Cardiac glycosides: digoxin (Lanoxin)
   j. Nitrates: isosorbide dinitrate (Isordil), nitroglycerin (Nitro-Bid)
   k. Diuretics: furosemide (Lasix), ethacrynic acid (Edecrin)
   l. Antiarrhythmics: quinidine (Cardioquin), procainamide HCl (Pronestyl)
   m. Anticoagulants: warfarin sodium (Coumadin)
   n. Antibiotics: pencillin G potassium (Pentids)
7. Medical nursing interventions/responsibilities
   a. Maintain diet
   b. Limit fluids
   c. Administer I.V. fluids
   d. Administer oxygen
   e. Assess cardiovascular and respiratory status
   f. Maintain semi-Fowler position
   g. Monitor and record VS, UO, I/O, hemodynamic variables, laboratory studies, EKG
   h. Administer medications
   i. Encourage ventilation of feelings about fear of death
   j. Assess pain
   k. Allay anxiety
   l. Assess peripheral edema
8. Patient/family teaching goals; the patient will:
   a. Keep follow-up appointments
   b. Stop smoking
   c. Maintain ideal weight
   d. State the action, side effects, and scheduling of medications
   e. Identify and reduce stress
   f. Recognize the signs and symptoms of CHF
   g. Adhere to activity limitations
   h. Avoid exposure to people with infections

     i. Alternate rest periods with activity
     j. Monitor self for infection
    k. Follow dietary recommendations and restrictions
     l. State need for antibiotic prophylaxis
    m. Test stools for occult blood

9. Possible medical complications
   a. Thrombus
   b. Embolus
   c. CHF
   d. Atrial fibrillation
10. Possible surgical interventions
   a. Valve replacement (see page 11)
   b. Open mitral commissurotomy (see page 11)

S. Mitral regurgitation: "insufficiency"

1. Definition: incomplete closure of the mitral valve
2. Possible etiology
   a. Congenital defect
   b. Rheumatic fever
   c. Trauma
   d. Papillary muscle dysfunction
   e. Bacterial endocarditis
3. Pathophysiology
   a. Valvular incompetence prevents complete closure of the mitral valve
   b. Incomplete valve closure permits backflow of blood to the left atrium
   c. Backflow of blood to the left atrium results in increased left atrial pressure, pulmonary hypertension, and left atrial hypertrophy
4. Possible clinical manifestations
   a. Shortness of breath
   b. Cough
   c. Fatigue
   d. Dyspnea on exertion
   e. Peripheral edema
   f. Atrial fibrillation
   g. Angina pectoris
   h. Orthopnea
   i. Hemoptysis
5. Possible diagnostic test findings
   a. CXR: enlargement of left atrium and left ventricle
   b. EKG: atrial fibrillation, left atrial hypertension, and left ventricular hypertrophy
   c. Echocardiogram: enlargement of left atrium, abnormal movement of mitral valve
   d. Cardiac catheterization: increased left atrial and left ventricular pressure
   e. Angiography: regurgitation

6. Medical management
   a. Diet therapy: low-sodium, restrict fluids
   b. I.V. therapy: heparin lock
   c. Oxygen therapy
   d. Position: semi-Fowler
   e. Monitoring: VS, UO, I/O, EKG, hemodynamic variables
   f. Laboratory studies: sodium, potassium, BUN, Cr, ABGs
   g. Treatments: Foley catheter
   h. Cardiac glycosides: digoxin (Lanoxin)
   i. Nitrates: isosorbide dinitrate (Isordil), nitroglycerin (Nitro-Bid)
   j. Diuretics: furosemide (Lasix), ethacrynic acid (Edecrin)
   k. Antiarrhythmics: quinidine (Cardioquin), procainamide HCl (Pronestyl)
   l. Anticoagulants: warfarin sodium (Coumadin)
7. Medical nursing interventions/responsibilities
   a. Maintain diet
   b. Limit fluids
   c. Administer I.V. fluids
   d. Administer oxygen
   e. Assess cardiovascular and respiratory status
   f. Maintain semi-Fowler position
   g. Monitor and record VS, UO, I/O, hemodynamic variables, laboratory studies, EKG
   h. Administer medications
   i. Encourage ventilation of feelings about fear of death
   j. Assess pain
   k. Assess peripheral edema
   l. Allay anxiety
8. Patient/family teaching goals; the patient will:
   a. Keep follow-up appointments
   b. Stop smoking
   c. Maintain ideal weight
   d. State the action, side effects, and scheduling of medications
   e. Identify and reduce stress
   f. Test stools for occult blood
   g. Adhere to activity limitations
   h. Avoid exposure to people with infections
   i. Alternate rest periods with activity
   j. Monitor self for infection
   k. Follow dietary recommendations and restrictions
   l. Differentiate between the pain of angina and the pain of MI
9. Possible medical complications
   a. Emboli
   b. Thrombus
   c. CHF
   d. Ruptured papillary muscle

10. Possible surgical interventions
    a. Mitral valve replacement (see page 11)
    b. Valvuloplasty (see page 11)

T. Aortic stenosis
1. Definition: narrowing of the aortic valve
2. Possible etiology
   a. Syphilis
   b. Rheumatic fever
   c. Atherosclerosis
   d. Congenital malformations
3. Pathophysiology
   a. Valvular tissue fibroses and calcifies, which narrows the valve opening and limits blood flow
   b. The narrowed opening results in incomplete emptying of the left ventricle, increased pressure, and hypertrophy of the left ventricle with decreased CO
   c. Congestion increases in the lungs, resulting in right ventricular failure
4. Possible clinical manifestations
   a. Angina pectoris
   b. Syncope
   c. Pulmonary hypertension
   d. Left-sided heart failure
   e. Fatigue
   f. Orthopnea
   g. PND
5. Possible diagnostic test findings
   a. CXR: aortic valve calcification, left ventricular enlargement
   b. EKG: left bundle branch block, 1st degree heart block, left ventricular hypertrophy
   c. Echocardiogram: thickened left ventricular wall, thickened aortic valve, abnormal movement of the aortic valve
   d. Cardiac catheterization: increased left ventricular pressure
6. Medical management
   a. Diet therapy: low-sodium, restrict fluids
   b. I.V. therapy: heparin lock
   c. Monitoring: VS, UO, I/O, EKG, hemodynamic variables
   d. Laboratory studies: sodium, potassium, BUN, Cr, ABGs
   e. Cardiac glycosides: digoxin (Lanoxin)
   f. Nitrates: isosorbide dinitrate (Isordil), nitroglycerin (Nitro-Bid)
   g. Diuretics: furosemide (Lasix), ethacrynic acid (Edecrin)
7. Medical nursing interventions/responsibilities
   a. Maintain diet
   b. Limit fluids
   c. Assess cardiovascular and respiratory status

   d. Monitor and record VS, UO, I/O, hemodynamic variables, laboratory studies, EKG
   e. Administer medications
   f. Encourage ventilation of feelings about fear of death
   g. Assess pain
   h. Allay anxiety
8. Patient/family teaching goals; the patient will:
   a. Keep follow-up appointments
   b. Stop smoking
   c. Maintain ideal weight
   d. State the action, side effects, and scheduling of medications
   e. Identify and reduce stress
   f. Recognize the signs and symptoms of CHF
   g. Adhere to activity limitations
   h. Alternate rest periods with activity
   i. Follow dietary recommendations and restrictions
9. Possible medical complications
   a. Sudden cardiac death
   b. CHF
   c. Pulmonary edema
10. Possible surgical interventions
    a. Aortic valve replacement (see page 11)
    b. Commissurotomy (see page 11)

U. Aortic regurgitation: "insufficiency"
1. Definition: incomplete closure of the aortic valve
2. Possible etiology
   a. Rheumatic fever
   b. Infective endocarditis
   c. Syphilis
   d. Atherosclerosis
   e. Congenital
3. Pathophysiology
   a. Incomplete closure of the valve results in retrograde flow of blood from the aorta to the left ventricle
   b. Pressure increases lead to left ventricular hypertrophy
4. Possible clinical manifestations
   a. Signs of left-sided heart failure
   b. Dyspnea on exertion
   c. Dizziness
   d. Neck pain
   e. Orthopnea
   f. Angina pectoris
   g. Tachycardia
   h. PND

5. Possible diagnostic test findings
   a. CXR: enlarged left ventricle, aortic valve calcification
   b. EKG: left ventricular hypertrophy, sinus tachycardia
   c. Echocardiogram: left ventricular enlargement, abnormal valve movement
   d. Cardiac catheterization: increased left atrial and left ventricular pressures
   e. Cardiac angiography: regurgitation
6. Medical managment
   a. Diet therapy: low-sodium, restrict fluids
   b. I.V. therapy: heparin lock
   c. Monitoring: VS, UO, I/O, EKG, hemodynamic variables
   d. Laboratory studies: ABGs, sodium, potassium, BUN, Cr
   e. Treatments: Foley catheter
   f. Antibiotics: penicillin G potassium (Pentids)
   g. Cardiac glycosides: digoxin (Lanoxin)
   h. Nitrates: isosorbide dinitrate (Isordil), nitroglycerin (Nitro-Bid)
   i. Diuretics: furosemide (Lasix), ethacrynic acid (Edecrin)
7. Medical nursing interventions/responsibilities
   a. Maintain diet
   b. Restrict fluids
   c. Administer I.V. fluids
   d. Assess cardiovascular and respiratory status
   e. Monitor and record VS, UO, I/O, hemodynamic variables, laboratory studies
   f. Assess pain
   g. Administer medications
   h. Encourage ventilation of feelings about fear of death
   i. Allay anxiety
8. Patient/family teaching goals; the patient will:
   a. Keep follow-up appointments
   b. Stop smoking
   c. Maintain ideal weight
   d. State the action, side effects, and scheduling of medications
   e. Identify and reduce stress
   f. Recognize the signs and symptoms of CHF
   g. Adhere to activity limitations
   h. Alternate rest periods with activity
   i. Monitor self for infection
   j. Follow dietary recommendations and restrictions
   k. Differentiate between the pain of angina and the pain of MI
9. Possible medical complications
   a. CHF
   b. Thrombus
   c. Embolus
   d. Infection

10. Possible surgical interventions
   a. Valvuloplasty (see page 11)
   b. Valve replacement (see page 11)

V. Peripheral vascular disease (PVD)
1. Definition
   a. Chronic inadequate blood flow in the lower extremities
   b. Types: arteriosclerosis obliterans, Raynaud's phenomena, Buerger's disease
2. Possible etiology
   a. Atherosclerosis
   b. Vasospasm
   c. Inflammation
3. Pathophysiology
   a. Artery walls thicken and lose elasticity, narrowing the diameter of the artery
   b. Decreased perfusion and the formation of blood clots cause blockage and ischemia
   c. Common sites are the femoral, popliteal, and iliac arteries and aorta
4. Possible clinical manifestations
   a. Intermittent claudication
   b. Pain at rest
   c. Trophic changes: thickened nails; absence of hair; taut, shiny skin
   d. Diminished or absent pulses
   e. Temperature changes in extremities
   f. Color changes: rubor, cyanosis, pallor
   g. Ulcerations
5. Possible diagnostic test findings
   a. Arteriography: location of obstructing plaque
   b. Doppler studies: decreased blood flow, decreased pressure
   c. Blood chemistry: increased lipids
6. Medical management
   a. Diet therapy: low-fat, low-calorie
   b. Activity: ad lib, active ROM, isometric exercises
   c. Monitoring: VS, I/O, neurovascular checks
   d. Laboratory studies: serum lipids, PTT, PT
   e. Treatments: bed cradle
   f. Analgesics: aspirin (Ecotrin)
   g. Vasodilators: papaverine HCl (Pavabid), isoxsuprine HCl (Vasodilan)
   h. Anticoagulants: warfarin sodium (Coumadin)
   i. Lipid reducers: cholestryamine (Questran), clofibrate (Atromid-S)
   j. Percutaneous transluminal angioplasty
7. Medical nursing interventions/responsibilities
   a. Maintain diet
   b. Assess cardiovascular status
   c. Monitor and record VS, UO, I/O, laboratory studies

    d. Administer medications
    e. Encourage ventilation of feelings about change in body image
    f. Assess peripheral circulation: pulses, color, temperature, sensation
    g. Encourage leg exercises and walking
    h. Provide daily foot care
8. Patient/family teaching goals; the patient will:
    a. Keep follow-up appointments
    b. Maintain regular exercise program
    c. Stop smoking
    d. Maintain ideal weight
    e. State the action, side effects, and scheduling of medications
    f. Recognize the signs and symptoms of decreased peripheral circulation
    g. Alternate rest periods with activity
    h. Monitor self for skin breakdown
    i. Follow dietary recommendations and restrictions
    j. Peform daily foot care
    k. Avoid injury to extremities
    l. Identify and reduce stress
    m. Avoid standing for long periods of time
    n. Avoid constrictive clothing
    o. Avoid crossing the legs at the knee when seated
    p. Avoid temperature extremes
9. Possible medical complications
    a. Gangrene
    b. Septicemia
    c. Decubitus ulcers
    d. Acute vascular occlusion
10. Possible surgical interventions
    a. Bypass grafting (see page 11)
    b. Endarterectomy (see page 85)
    c. Sympathectomy
    d. Amputation (see page 50)
    e. Embolectomy (see page 232)

W. Thrombophlebitis
1. Definition: inflammation of venous wall with clot formation
2. Possible etiology
    a. Venous stasis: varicose veins, pregnancy, CHF, prolonged bed rest
    b. Hypercoagulability: cancer, blood dyscrasias, oral contraceptives
    c. Injury to the venous wall: I.V. injections, fractures, antibiotics
3. Pathophysiology
    a. Venous stasis, hypercoagulability of the blood, and injury to the venous wall result in the massing of red blood cells in a fibrin network
    b. As the thrombus enlarges, it causes an obstruction, resulting in venous insufficiency
    c. Common sites are deep veins and superficial veins

4. Possible clinical manifestations
   a. Superficial: red, warm skin, tender to touch
   b. Deep: edema, positive Homans' sign, tender to touch, cramping pain
5. Possible diagnostic test findings
   a. Venography: venous-filling defects
   b. Ultrasound: decreased blood flow
   c. Phlebography: venous-filling defects
   d. Hematology: increased WBC
6. Medical management
   a. Position: elevation of extremity
   b. Activity: bed rest, active and passive ROM, isometric exercises
   c. Monitoring: VS, neurovascular checks
   d. Laboratory studies: WBC, PT, PTT
   e. Treatments: antiembolitic stockings; warm, moist compresses
   f. Anticoagulants: warfarin sodium (Coumadin), heparin sodium (Lipo-Hepin)
   g. Exercise prescription
   h. Fibrinolytic agents: streptokinase
   i. Vasodilators: papaverine HCl (Pavabid), isoxsuprine HCl (Vasodilan)
   j. Anti-inflammatory agents: aspirin (Ecotrin)
7. Medical nursing interventions/responsibilities
   a. Assess cardiovascular status
   b. Maintain bed rest with elevation of extremities
   c. Monitor and record VS, neurovascular checks, laboratory studies
   d. Administer medications
   e. Assess Homans' sign
   f. Assess for bleeding
   g. Apply warm, moist compresses
   h. Measure girth of thighs and calves
8. Patient/family teaching goals; the patient will:
   a. Keep follow-up appointments
   b. Maintain regular exercise program
   c. Stop smoking
   d. Maintain ideal weight
   e. State the action, side effects, and scheduling of medications
   f. Identify and reduce stress
   g. Recognize the signs and symptoms of bleeding
   h. Avoid prolonged sitting and standing
   i. Avoid constrictive clothing
   j. Avoid crossing legs when seated
   k. Avoid oral contraceptives
9. Possible medical complications
   a. Pulmonary embolism
   b. CVA

10. Possible surgical interventions
    a. Vena cava filter (plication of inferior vena cava) (see page 233)
    b. Vein ligation and stripping
    c. Thrombectomy

X. Bacterial endocarditis
1. Definition: inflammation and infection of the endocardial lining of the heart
2. Possible etiology
    a. Bacterial infection: B-hemolytic streptococcus, *Staphylococcus aureus*
    b. Rheumatic heart disease
    c. Dental extractions
    d. Invasive monitoring
3. Pathophysiology
    a. Bacteria form colonies on endocardial lining of the valves and destroy the valve leaflets
    b. Blood flow is disrupted, resulting in murmurs
    c. Vegetations then seed the bloodstream with bacteria
4. Possible clinical manifestations
    a. Elevated temperature
    b. Heart murmur
    c. Diaphoresis
    d. Malaise
    e. Dyspnea
    f. Tachycardia
    g. Clubbing of fingers and toes
    h. Petechiae
    i. Night sweats
    j. Splinter hemorrhages in nailbeds
5. Possible diagnostic test findings
    a. Blood cultures: positive for specific organism
    b. Hematology: increased WBC, ESR; decreased Hct
    c. Echocardiography: valvular damage, vegetations
6. Medical management
    a. I.V. therapy: hydration, heparin lock
    b. Oxygen therapy
    c. Activity: bed rest
    d. Monitoring: VS, UO, I/O, neurovascular checks
    e. Laboratory studies: blood cultures, WBC, Hct
    f. Antibiotics: penicillin G potassium (Pentids)
    g. Fluids: encourage intake
    h. Antipyretics: aspirin (Ecotrin)
    i. Anticoagulants: warfarin sodium (Coumadin)
7. Medical nursing interventions/responsibilities
    a. Force fluids
    b. Administer I.V. fluids

      c. Administer oxygen
      d. Assess cardiovascular status
      e. Monitor and record VS, UO, I/O, laboratory studies
      f. Administer medications
      g. Encourage ventilation of feelings about fear of dying
      h. Allay anxiety
  8. Patient/family teaching goals; the patient will:
      a. Keep follow-up appointments
      b. Maintain regular exercise program
      c. Stop smoking
      d. Maintain ideal weight
      e. State the action, side effects, and scheduling of medications
      f. Identify and reduce stress
      g. Recognize the signs and symptoms of endocarditis
      h. Follow activity limitations
      i. Avoid exposure to people with infections
      j. Alternate rest periods with activity
      k. Monitor self for infection, particularly after dental and gynecologic exams
      l. State need for antibiotic prophylaxis
      m. Wear medical identification bracelet
  9. Possible medical complications
      a. Embolism
      b. CHF
      c. Mycotic aneurysm
 10. Possible surgical interventions: valve replacement (see page 11)

Y. Abdominal aortic aneurysm

  1. Definition: dilation or localized weakness in the medial layer of an artery
  2. Possible etiology
      a. Atherosclerosis
      b. Congenital defect
      c. Trauma
      d. Syphilis
      e. Hypertension
      f. Infection
  3. Pathophysiology
      a. Degenerative changes caused by atherosclerosis result in a weakness in the medial layer
      b. Force of blood pressure continues to weaken the wall and results in outpouching of the artery
      c. Types: saccular, fusiform, dissecting, false
  4. Possible clinical manifestations
      a. Asymptomatic
      b. Lower abdominal, low back pain
      c. Abdominal mass left of midline

d. Abdominal pulsations
e. Bruit
f. Diminished femoral pulses
g. Systolic blood pressure in legs lower than systolic blood pressure in arms

5. Possible diagnostic test findings
   a. CXR: presence of aneurysm
   b. EKG: differentiation of aneurysm from MI
   c. Echocardiography: presence of aneurysm
   d. Aortography: presence of aneurysm

6. Medical management
   a. Activity: bed rest
   b. Monitoring: VS, UO, I/O, neurovascular checks
   c. Analgesics: oxycodone HCl (Tylox)
   d. Beta-adrenergic blockers: propranolol (Inderal)
   e. Antihypertensives: methyldopa (Aldomet), hydralazine (Apresoline), prazosin (Minipress)

7. Medical nursing interventions/responsibilities
   a. Assess cardiovascular status
   b. Monitor and record VS, UO, I/O, neurovascular checks, laboratory studies
   c. Administer medications
   d. Encourage ventilation of feelings about fear of death
   e. Assess pain
   f. Assess peripheral circulation: pulses, temperature, color, sensation
   g. Allay anxiety
   h. Assess for signs of shock
   i. Palpate abdomen

8. Patient/family teaching goals; the patient will:
   a. Keep follow-up appointments
   b. Stop smoking
   c. State the action, side effects, and scheduling of medications
   d. Identify and reduce stress
   e. Recognize the signs and symptoms of decreased peripheral circulation
   f. Adhere to activity limitations
   g. Alternate rest periods with activity
   h. Maintain a quiet environment

9. Possible medical complications: rupture of aneurysm
10. Possible surgical interventions: resection of aneurysm (see page 12)

Points to Remember

Complaints of chest pain have increased significance in patients with a peripheral vascular problem.

A unilateral finding in the assessment of peripheral circulation has greater significance than bilateral findings.

The impact of cardiovascular disease can be reduced by altering modifiable risk factors.

The focus of nursing management in cardiovascular disorders is to increase blood supply and oxygenation to tissues.

Alterations in cardiac output affect every system in the body.

Glossary

Bruit — sound of abnormal blood flow heard on auscultation.

Intermittent claudication — calf pain that is precipitated by walking and relieved with rest.

Jugular venous distention — distended neck veins that indirectly indicate increased central venous pressure.

Orthopnea — respiratory distress that is relieved by sitting upright.

Paroxysmal nocturnal dyspnea — respiratory distress that occurs after lying in a recumbent position for several hours.

Musculoskeletal System

Learning Objectives

After studying this section, the reader should be able to:

• Describe the psychosocial impact of musculoskeletal system disorders.

• Differentiate between modifiable and nonmodifiable risk factors in the development of a musculoskeletal system disorder.

• List three potential and three actual nursing diagnoses for the patient who has a musculoskeletal system disorder.

• Identify the medical and surgical nursing interventions/ responsibilities for the patient who has a musculoskeletal system disorder.

• Write three teaching goals for the patient who has a musculoskeletal system disorder.

II. Musculoskeletal System

A. Anatomy and physiology
1. Skeleton
   a. Bones (206) are described as long, short, flat, and irregular
   b. Bones store calcium, magnesium, and phosphorus
   c. Bone marrow produces red blood cells (RBC)
   d. Bones work with muscles to provide support, locomotion, and protection of internal organs
2. Skeletal muscles
   a. These muscles provide body movement and posture by tightening and shortening
   b. They attach to bones by tendons
   c. Contraction begins with the stimulus of a muscle fiber by a motor neuron
   d. Energy for muscle contraction comes from hydrolysis of adenosine triphosphate (ATP) into adenosine diphosphate (ADP) and phosphate
   e. Residual amount of muscle contraction is known as muscle tone
   f. Muscle relaxation results from breakdown of acetylcholine by cholinesterase
3. Ligaments
   a. These tough bands of collagen fibers connect bones to bones
   b. They encircle a joint to add strength and stability
4. Tendons
   a. Nonelastic collagen cords
   b. Function: connect muscles to bones
5. Joints
   a. Articulation of two bone surfaces
   b. Degree of joint movement is called range of motion (ROM)
   c. Function: provide stabilization and permit locomotion
6. Synovium
   a. Membrane lining the inner surfaces of a joint; secretes synovial fluid and antibodies
   b. Function: in conjunction with cartilage, reduces friction of joints
7. Cartilage
   a. Serves as a smooth surface for articulating bones and absorbing shock to joints
   b. Atrophies with absence of weight bearing or limited ROM
8. Bursa
   a. Fluid-filled sac that facilitates motion of structures that move against each other
   b. Padding to reduce friction

B. Physical assessment findings
1. Subjective data that often accompany musculoskeletal disorders
   a. Pain
   b. Numbness

    c. Joint stiffness
    d. Swelling
    e. Fatigue
    f. Fever
    g. Difficulty with movement
2. Objective data to evaluate in musculoskeletal disorders
    a. Vital signs (VS)
    b. Inflammation
    c. Edema
    d. Skin integrity
    e. Skeletal deformity
    f. ROM
    g. Posture
    h. Muscle strength, size, and tone
    i. Skin color and temperature
    j. Paresthesia
    k. Nodules
    l. Erythema
    m. Tophi
    n. Peripheral pulses
    o. Muscle spasms
    p. Pain
    q. Ambulation
    r. Skin temperature

C. Diagnostic tests and procedures used to evaluate musculoskeletal disorders

1. Electromyography (EMG)
    a. Definition/purpose: noninvasive test that graphically records the electrical activity of the muscle at rest and during contraction
    b. Nursing interventions/responsibilities: before procedure, advise the patient that he will be asked to flex and relax muscles during the procedure; after procedure, administer analgesics as ordered
2. Arthroscopy
    a. Definition/purpose: direct visualization of a joint using an arthroscope after injection of local anesthesia
    b. Nursing interventions/responsibilities: before procedure, administer prophylactic antibiotics as ordered; after procedure, maintain pressure dressing to site; monitor neurovascular status; apply ice to knee; limit weight bearing; administer analgesics as ordered
3. Arthrocentesis
    a. Definition/purpose: needle aspiration of synovial fluid from a joint under local anesthesia to examine specimen or remove synovial fluid
    b. Nursing interventions/responsibilities: before procedure, administer prophylactic antibiotics as ordered; after procedure, maintain pressure dressing on site; monitor neurovascular status; apply ice to knee; limit weight bearing; administer analgesics as ordered

4. Bone scan
   a. Definition/purpose: visual imaging of bone metabolism after I.V. injection of radioisotope
   b. Nursing interventions/responsibilities: before procedure, assess patient's ability to lie still during the scan
5. Myelogram
   a. Definition/purpose: injection of radiopaque dye by lumbar puncture to visualize the subarachnoid space, spinal cord, and vertebral bodies under fluoroscopy
   b. Nursing interventions/responsibilities: before procedure, assess allergies to iodine, seafood, and radiopaque dyes; inform patient that he may feel flushing of the face and throat irritation; after procedure, maintain flat bed rest as ordered; assess insertion site for bleeding; monitor neurovital signs; force fluids
6. X-ray examination
   a. Definition/purpose: radiographic picture of bones and joints
   b. Nursing interventions/responsibilities: use caution while moving patients with a suspected fracture
7. Blood chemistry
   a. Definition/purpose: laboratory analysis of blood sample for potassium, sodium, calcium, phosphorus, glucose, bicarbonate, blood urea nitrogen (BUN), creatinine (Cr), protein, albumin, osmolality, creatine phosphokinase (CPK), serum glutamic-oxalacetic transaminase (SGOT), aldolase, rheumatoid factor, complement fixation, lupus erythematosus cell preparation (LE prep), antinuclear antibody (ANA), anti-DNA, and C-reactive protein
   b. Nursing interventions/responsibilities: before procedure, withhold food and fluid as ordered; after procedure, monitor site for bleeding
8. Hematologic studies
   a. Definition/purpose: laboratory analysis of blood sample for white blood cells (WBC), RBC, platelets, prothrombin time (PT), partial thromboplastin time (PTT), erythrocyte sedimentation rate (ESR), hemoglobin (Hgb), and hematocrit (Hct)
   b. Nursing interventions/responsibilities: assess site for bleeding, note current drug therapy

D. **Possible psychosocial impact of musculoskeletal disorders**
   1. Developmental impact
      a. Decreased self-esteem
      b. Fear of rejection
      c. Change in body image
      d. Embarrassment from change in body structure and function
      e. Dependency

2. Economic impact
    a. Disruption or loss of employment
    b. Cost of vocational retraining
    c. Cost of hospitalizations
    d. Cost of home health care
    e. Cost of special equipment
3. Occupational and recreational impact
    a. Restrictions in work activity
    b. Change in leisure activity
    c. Restrictions in physical activity
4. Social impact
    a. Social isolation
    b. Changes in role performance

E. Possible risk factors for development of musculoskeletal system disorders
1. Modifiable risk factors
    a. Occupations that require heavy lifting or use of machinery
    b. Occupational or recreational activities that include repetitive motion of joints
    c. Vegetarian diets
    d. Immobility
    e. Medication history
    f. Stress
    g. Contact sports
    h. Obesity
2. Nonmodifiable risk factors
    a. Aging process
    b. Menopause
    c. Family history of musculoskeletal illness
    d. History of musculoskeletal injury
    e. History of immune disorders

F. Possible nursing diagnoses for the patient with musculoskeletal system disorders
1. Actual nursing diagnoses
    a. Impaired physical mobility
    b. Alteration in tissue perfusion: peripheral
    c. Impairment of skin integrity
    d. Alteration in comfort: pain
    e. Self-care deficit: toileting
    f. Self-care deficit: feeding
    g. Self-care deficit: bathing
2. Potential nursing diagnoses
    a. Sexual dysfunction
    b. Powerlessness

     c. Alteration in bowel elimination: constipation
     d. Disturbance in self-concept: body image
     e. Social isolation

G. Surgical intervention: joint surgery

  1. Definition
     a. Arthrodesis: removal of cartilage from joint surfaces to surgically fuse a joint into a functional position
     b. Synovectomy: removal of the synovial membrane from a joint using an arthroscope, to reduce pain
     c. Total joint replacement (arthroplasty): surgical replacement of a joint using a metal, plastic, or porous coated prosthesis
  2. Preoperative surgical nursing interventions/responsibilities
     a. Complete patient and family preoperative teaching: assess understanding of surgical procedure; explain operating room (OR), recovery room (RR), preoperative, and postoperative routine; demonstrate postoperative turning, coughing, and deep breathing (TCDB), splinting, leg exercises, and ROM; explain postoperative need for drainage tubes, surgical dressings, oxygen therapy, I.V. therapy, and pain control
     b. Complete preoperative check list
     c. Administer preoperative medications
     d. Allay patient and family anxiety about surgery
     e. Document patient history and physical assessment data base
     f. Administer antibiotics
  3. Postoperative surgical nursing interventions/responsibilities
     a. Assess cardiac and respiratory status
     b. Assess pain and administer postoperative analgesic
     c. Progress diet as tolerated
     d. Administer I.V. fluids and transfusion therapy
     e. Allay anxiety
     f. Assess surgical dressing and change as directed
     g. Reinforce TCDB
     h. Maintain semi-Fowler position
     i. Assess for return of peristalsis
     j. Provide pulmonary toilet: incentive spirometry
     k. Maintain activity: as tolerated, active and passive ROM, isometric exercises
     l. Monitor VS, urinary output (UO), intake and output (I/O), laboratory studies, neurovascular checks
     m. Monitor and maintain position and patency of drainage tubes: wound drainage
     n. Encourage ventilation of feelings about change in mobility
     o. Assess movement limitations
     p. Elevate affected extremity

    q. Arthrodesis: provide routine cast care
    r. Total knee replacement: maintain continuous passive motion (CPM), apply knee immobilizer before getting out of bed (OOB)
    s. Total hip replacement: maintain hips in abduction, limit hip flexion to 90° when sitting

4. Possible surgical complications
    a. Infection
    b. Hemorrhage

5. Patient/family postoperative teaching goals; the patient will:
    a. Keep follow-up appointments
    b. Maintain regular exercise program
    c. Maintain ideal weight
    d. State the action, side effects, and scheduling of medications
    e. Recognize the signs and symptoms of infection
    f. Avoid jogging, jumping, lifting
    g. Complete daily incision care
    h. Arthrodesis: maintain cast care
    i. Use ambulation assists: crutches, cane, walker
    j. Total hip replacement: avoid sitting in low chairs and crossing legs

H. Surgical intervention: external fixation

1. Definition: fracture immobilization in which a series of transfixing pins is inserted through bone above and below the fracture and attached to a rigid external metal frame
2. Preoperative surgical nursing interventions/responsibilities
    a. Complete patient and family preoperative teaching: assess understanding of surgical procedure; explain OR, RR, preoperative, and postoperative routine; demonstrate postoperative TCDB, splinting, leg exercises, and ROM; explain postoperative need for drainage tubes, surgical dressings, oxygen therapy, I.V. therapy, and pain control
    b. Complete preoperative check list
    c. Administer preoperative medications
    d. Allay patient and family anxiety about surgery
    e. Document patient history and physical assessment data base
    f. Monitor for fracture complications
    g. Maintain position of affected extremity with sandbags and pillows
    h. Maintain traction or splint
3. Postoperative surgical nursing interventions/responsibilities
    a. Assess pain and administer postoperative analgesic
    b. Progress diet as tolerated
    c. Administer I.V. fluids
    d. Allay anxiety
    e. Reinforce TCDB
    f. Maintain semi-Fowler position
    g. Assess for return of peristalsis

h. Provide pulmonary toilet: incentive spirometry
i. Maintain activity: as tolerated, active and passive ROM, isometric exercises, quad sets
j. Monitor VS, UO, I/O, laboratory studies, neurovascular checks
k. Encourage ventilation of feelings about change in body image
l. Monitor for infection of wound and pin sites
m. Provide pin care
n. Maintain balanced supension traction
o. Do not adjust clamps

4. Possible surgical complications
    a. Infection of wound and pin sites
    b. Osteomyelitis
    c. Hemorrhage
    d. Chronic pain

5. Patient/family postoperative teaching goals; the patient will:
    a. Keep follow-up appointments
    b. Maintain regular exercise program and physical therapy
    c. Maintain fixator as set
    d. Maintain ideal weight
    e. State the action, side effects, and scheduling of medications
    f. Recognize the signs and symptoms of soft tissue and bone infection
    g. Adhere to activity limitations
    h. Complete daily wound and pin care
    i. Use ambulation assists: crutches, walker, cane

I. Surgical intervention: amputation

1. Definition
    a. Surgical removal of all or part of a limb
    b. Types: closed (flap), open (guillotine)

2. Preoperative surgical nursing interventions/responsibilities
    a. Complete patient and family preoperative teaching: assess understanding of surgical procedure; explain OR, RR, preoperative and postoperative routine; demonstrate postoperative TCDB, splinting, leg exercises, and ROM; explain postoperative need for drainage tubes, surgical dressings, oxygen therapy, I.V. therapy, and pain control
    b. Complete preoperative check list
    c. Administer preoperative medications
    d. Allay patient and family anxiety about surgery
    e. Document patient history and physical assessment data base
    f. Administer antibiotics
    g. Prepare the patient for the possibility of phantom limb sensation or phantom pain

3. Postoperative surgical nursing interventions/responsibilities
    a. Assess cardiac and respiratory status
    b. Assess pain and administer postoperative analgesic
    c. Progress diet as tolerated

       d. Administer I.V. fluids and transfusion therapy
       e. Allay anxiety
       f. Assess surgical dressing and change as directed
       g. Reinforce TCDB
       h. Maintain semi-Fowler position
       i. Assess for return of peristalsis
       j. Provide pulmonary toilet: incentive spirometry
       k. Maintain activity: as tolerated, active and passive ROM, isometric exercises
       l. Monitor VS, UO, I/O, laboratory studies, neurovascular checks
       m. Monitor and maintain position and patency of drainage tubes: wound drainage
       n. Encourage ventilation of feelings about change in body image, phantom limb sensation and phantom pain, depression
       o. Administer antibiotics
       p. Elevate lower extremity amputation for 24 hours only
       q. Rewrap stump before getting patient out of bed
       r. Prevent hip flexion
       s. Assess stump for bleeding, infection, and edema
       t. Maintain rigid dressing for stump prosthesis
       u. Irrigate wound and change stump dressing as directed
       v. Reinforce physical therapy attendance
  4. Possible surgical complications
       a. Hemorrhage
       b. Infection
       c. Contractures
       d. Skin breakdown
  5. Patient/family postoperative teaching goals; the patient will:
       a. Keep follow-up appointments
       b. Maintain regular exercise program
       c. Stop smoking
       d. Maintain ideal weight
       e. State the action, side effects, and scheduling of medications
       f. Recognize the signs and symptoms of infection and skin breakdown
       g. Complete daily stump care
       h. Use specialized appliances: prosthesis
       i. Maintain stump conditioning program
       j. Avoid use of powder or lotion on stump
       k. Demonstrate wrapping of the stump
       l. Use ambulation assists: crutches, cane, walker
       m. Protect stump from injury

J. Surgical intervention: release of transverse carpal ligament
  1. Definition: surgical ligation of the transverse carpal ligament to relieve compression of the median nerve in the carpal canal of the wrist

2. Postoperative surgical nursing interventions/responsibilities
   a. Complete patient and family preoperative teaching: assess understanding of surgical procedure; explain OR, RR, preoperative and postoperative routine; demonstrate postoperative TCDB, splinting, leg exercises, and ROM; explain postoperative need for drainage tubes, surgical dressings, oxygen therapy, I.V. therapy, and pain control
   b. Complete preoperative check list
   c. Administer preoperative medications
   d. Allay patient and family anxiety about surgery
   e. Document patient history and physical assessment data base
   f. Maintain position of comfort with a splint
3. Postoperative surgical nursing interventions/responsibilities
   a. Assess pain and administer postoperative analgesic
   b. Progress diet as tolerated
   c. Administer I.V. fluids
   d. Allay anxiety
   e. Assess surgical dressing and change as directed
   f. Reinforce TCDB
   g. Maintain semi-Fowler position
   h. Assess for return of peristalsis
   i. Provide pulmonary toilet: incentive spirometry
   j. Maintain activity: as tolerated, active and passive ROM, isometric exercises
   k. Monitor VS, UO, I/O, laboratory studies, neurovascular checks
   l. Elevate hand and apply ice
   m. Administer steroids
   n. Administer antibiotics
   o. Assist with activities of daily living (ADL)
   p. Prevent injury to affected hand
   q. Apply splint
   r. Reinforce immobilization of affected hand
4. Possible surgical complications
   a. Infection
   b. Paralysis of hand
5. Patient/family postoperative teaching goals; the patient will:
   a. Keep follow-up appointments
   b. Maintain regular exercise program and active ROM of affected hand
   c. Stop smoking
   d. Maintain ideal weight
   e. State the action, side effects, and scheduling of medications
   f. Recognize the signs and symptoms of infection
   g. Avoid heavy lifting
   h. Complete daily incision care
   i. Use specialized appliances: splint
   j. Elevate affected hand
   k. Monitor return of sensation and motor function in affected hand

K. Surgical intervention: open reduction internal fixation (ORIF)
1. Definition: surgical reduction and stabilization of a fracture using orthopedic devices or hardware such as Austin-Moore prosthesis, Smith-Petersen nail, Jewett nail, intramedullary nails, and compression screws
2. Postoperative surgical nursing interventions/responsibilities
   a. Complete patient and family preoperative teaching: assess understanding of surgical procedure; explain OR, RR, preoperative and postoperative routine; demonstrate postoperative TCDB, splinting, leg exercises, and ROM; explain postoperative need for drainage tubes, surgical dressings, oxygen therapy, I.V. therapy, and pain control
   b. Complete preoperative check list
   c. Administer preoperative medications
   d. Allay patient and family anxiety about surgery
   e. Document patient history and physical assessment data base
   f. Monitor for fracture complications
   g. Maintain position of affected extremity with sandbags and pillows
   h. Maintain traction or splint
3. Postoperative surgical nursing interventions/responsibilities
   a. Assess cardiac and respiratory status
   b. Assess pain and administer postoperative analgesic
   c. Progress diet as tolerated
   d. Administer I.V. fluids and transfusion therapy
   e. Allay anxiety
   f. Assess surgical dressing and change as directed
   g. Reinforce TCDB
   h. Maintain semi-Fowler position: no higher than 30°
   i. Assess for return of peristalsis
   j. Provide pulmonary toilet: incentive spirometry
   k. Maintain activity: bed rest, active and passive ROM, isometric exercises, progressive ambulation
   l. Monitor VS, UO, I/O, laboratory studies, neurovascular checks
   m. Monitor and maintain position and patency of drainage tubes: Hemovac, Foley
   n. Use abductor pillow
   o. Turn to unaffected side
   p. Maintain high-fiber, low-calcium diet with increased fluid intake
   q. Apply antiembolitic stockings
   r. Administer anticoagulants
   s. Administer antibiotics
4. Possible surgical complications
   a. Osteomyelitis
   b. Hemorrhage
   c. Thrombophlebitis
   d. Pneumonia
   e. Avascular necrosis

5. Patient/family postoperative teaching goals; the patient will:
    a. Keep follow-up appointments
    b. Maintain regular exercise program
    c. Maintain ideal weight
    d. State the action, side effects, and scheduling of medications
    e. Recognize the signs and symptoms of infection
    f. Avoid sitting in low chairs, crossing legs, jogging, jumping, lifting
    g. Complete daily incision care
    h. Use ambulation assists after fixation with Austin-Moore prosthesis: walkers, crutches, canes
    i. Apply antiembolitic stockings

L. Surgical intervention: laminectomy
1. Definition: surgical excision of vertebral posterior arch
2. Preoperative surgical nursing interventions/responsibilities
    a. Complete patient and family preoperative teaching: assess understanding of surgical procedure; explain OR, RR, preoperative and postoperative routine; demonstrate postoperative TCDB, splinting, leg exercises, and ROM; explain postoperative need for drainage tubes, surgical dressings, oxygen therapy, I.V. therapy, and pain control
    b. Complete preoperative check list
    c. Administer preoperative medications
    d. Allay patient and family anxiety about surgery
    e. Document patient history and physical assessment data base
    f. Teach patient logrolling technique
    g. Administer antibiotics
3. Postoperative surgical nursing interventions/responsibilities
    a. Assess neurological and neurovascular status
    b. Assess pain and administer postoperative analgesic
    c. Progress diet as tolerated
    d. Administer I.V. fluids
    e. Allay anxiety
    f. Assess surgical dressing for drainage: cerebrospinal fluid (CSF), blood
    g. Reinforce TCDB
    h. Maintain flat position
    i. Assess for return of peristalsis
    j. Provide pulmonary toilet: incentive spirometry
    k. Maintain activity: active and passive ROM, isometric exercises
    l. Monitor VS, UO, I/O, laboratory studies, neurovascular checks
    m. Turn patient by logrolling
    n. Prevent flexion of the neck: cervical laminectomy
    o. Administer muscle relaxants
    p. Administer corticosteroids
4. Possible surgical complications
    a. Urinary retention
    b. Motor and sensory deficits

    c. Infection

    d. Muscle spasm

    e. Paralytic ileus

5. Patient/family postoperative teaching goals; the patient will:

    a. Keep follow-up appointments

    b. Maintain regular exercise program

    c. Stop smoking

    d. Maintain ideal weight

    e. State the action, side effects, and scheduling of medications

    f. Recognize the signs and symptoms of infection and motor or sensory deficits

    g. Adhere to activity limitations: no lifting, tub baths, driving, repetitive bending, stooping, sitting for prolonged periods of time

    h. Complete daily incision care

    i. Alternate rest periods with activity

    j. Wear supportive brace

    k. Complete low back exercises daily

    l. Sleep in side-lying position with hips and knees flexed

    m. Sleep on firm mattress

M. Surgical intervention: spinal fusion

1. Definition: stabilization of spinous processes with bone chips from iliac crest or Harrington rod metallic implant

2. Preoperative surgical nursing interventions/responsibilities

    a. Complete patient and family preoperative teaching: assess understanding of surgical procedure; explain OR, RR, preoperative and postoperative routine; demonstrate postoperative TCDB, splinting, leg exercises, and ROM; explain postoperative need for drainage tubes, surgical dressings, oxygen therapy, I.V. therapy, and pain control

    b. Complete preoperative check list

    c. Administer preoperative medications

    d. Allay patient and family anxiety about surgery

    e. Document patient history and physical assessment data base

    f. Administer antibiotics

    g. Teach patient logrolling technique

3. Postoperative surgical nursing interventions/responsibilities

    a. Assess cardiac, respiratory, and neurologic status

    b. Assess pain and administer postoperative analgesic

    c. Progress diet as tolerated

    d. Administer I.V. fluids

    e. Allay anxiety

    f. Assess surgical dressing and change as directed

    g. Reinforce TCDB

    h. Maintain supine position

    i. Assess for return of peristalsis

    j. Provide pulmonary toilet: incentive spirometry

      k. Maintain activity: active and passive ROM, isometric exercises
      l. Monitor VS, UO, I/O, laboratory studies
      m. Assess neurovascular status: color, temperature, pulses, movement, and sensation of extremities
      n. Administer antipyretics
      o. Administer antibiotics
      p. Administer corticosteroids
      q. Turn patient every 2 hours using logrolling technique
      r. Administer muscle relaxants
   4. Possible surgical complications
      a. Urinary retention
      b. Infection
      c. Muscle spasm
      d. Motor and sensory deficits
      e. Paralytic ileus
   5. Patient/family postoperative teaching goals; the patient will:
      a. Keep follow-up appointments
      b. Maintain regular exercise program
      c. Stop smoking
      d. Maintain ideal weight
      e. State the action, side effects, and scheduling of medications
      f. Recognize the signs and symptoms of infection, motor and sensory deficits
      g. Avoid lifting, repetitive bending, driving, tub baths, stooping, sitting for prolonged periods
      h. Complete daily incision care
      i. Maintain schedule of ambulation
      j. State spinal flexion limitations
      k. Complete low back exercises daily
      l. Sleep in side-lying position with hips and knees flexed
      m. Sleep on firm mattress

N. Rheumatoid arthritis

   1. Definition: systemic inflammatory disease that affects the synovial lining of the joints
   2. Possible etiology
      a. Unknown
      b. Autoimmune disease
      c. Genetic
   3. Pathophysiology
      a. Inflammation of synovial membranes is followed by pannus formation and destruction of cartilage, bone, and ligaments
      b. Pannus is replaced by fibrotic tissue and calcification, which causes subluxation of the joint

4. Possible clinical manifestations
   a. Fatigue
   b. Anorexia
   c. Malaise
   d. Elevated body temperature
   e. Painful, swollen joints
   f. Limited ROM
   g. Subcutaneous nodules
   h. "Mirror image" of affected joints: symmetrical joint swelling
   i. Morning stiffness
   j. Paresthesias of hands and feet
   k. Crepitus
   l. Pericarditis
   m. Splenomegaly
   n. Leukopenia
   o. Enlarged lymph nodes
5. Possible diagnostic test findings
   a. X-rays: joint space narrowing, bone erosions
   b. Hematology: increased ESR, WBC, platelets
   c. Gamma globulin: increased IgM, IgG
   d. Synovial fluid analysis: increased WBC, decreased viscosity, opaque
   e. Latex fixation test: positive rheumatoid factor
6. Medical management
   a. Activity: as tolerated
   b. Monitoring: VS, UO, I/O
   c. Analgesics: aspirin (Ecotrin)
   d. Nonsteroidal anti-inflammatory drugs (NSAID): indomethacin (Indocin), ibuprofen (Motrin), sulindac (Clinoril), piroxicam (Feldene)
   e. Glucocorticoids: prednisone (Deltasone), hydrocortisone (Cortef)
   f. Antacids: magnesium and aluminum hydroxide (Maalox), aluminum hydroxide gel (Gelusil)
   g. Gold therapy: sodium thiomalate (Myochrysine)
   h. Physical therapy
   i. Heat therapy/cold therapy
   j. Plasmapheresis
   k. Laboratory studies: ESR, WBC
7. Medical nursing interventions/responsibilities
   a. Assess neuromuscular status
   b. Maintain joints in position of extension
   c. Monitor and record VS, UO, I/O, laboratory studies
   d. Administer medications
   e. Encourage ventilation of feelings about change in body image and self-esteem
   f. Provide skin care

     g. Minimize environmental stress
     h. Assess joints for swelling, pain, and redness
     i. Provide ROM
     j. Provide heat therapy as ordered: warm compresses, paraffin dips
  8. Patient/family teaching goals; the patient will:
     a. Keep follow-up appointments
     b. Maintain regular exercise program
     c. Maintain ideal weight
     d. State the action, side effects, and scheduling of medications
     e. Identify and reduce stress
     f. Recognize the signs and symptoms of skin breakdown
     g. Adhere to activity limitations
     h. Alternate rest periods with activity
     i. Promote a safe environment
     j. Seek help from community agencies and resources
     k. Alter ADL to compensate for limited ROM
     l. Complete daily skin and foot care
     m. Avoid precipitating factors: cold, stress, infection
     n. Use assistive devices for ADL
     o. Use good body mechanics
     p. Avoid unproven remedies
  9. Possible medical complications: carpal tunnel syndrome
 10. Possible surgical interventions
     a. Joint replacement (see page 48)
     b. Synovectomy (see page 48)

O. Osteoarthritis (degenerative joint disease)

  1. Definition: degeneration of articular cartilage, usually affecting weight-bearing joints: spine, knees, hips
  2. Possible etiology
     a. Aging process
     b. Obesity
     c. Joint trauma
     d. Congenital abnormalities
  3. Pathophysiology
     a. Cartilage softens with age, narrowing the joint space
     b. Normal "wear and tear" thins and erodes cartilage
     c. Cartilage flakes enter the synovial lining, which fibroses, thus limiting joint movement
  4. Possible clinical manifestations
     a. Pain relieved by resting joints
     b. Joint stiffness
     c. Heberden's nodules
     d. Limited ROM
     e. Crepitation

  f. Increased pain in damp, cold weather
  g. Enlarged, edematous joints
  h. Smooth, taut, shiny skin
 5. Possible diagnostic test findings
  a. X-rays: joint deformity, narrowing of joint space, bone spurs
  b. Arthroscopy: bone spurs, narrowing of joint space
  c. Hematology: increased ESR
 6. Medical management
  a. Diet therapy: low-calorie
  b. Activity: as tolerated
  c. Monitoring: VS, UO, I/O
  d. Heat/cold therapy
  e. Exercise program: isometrics
  f. Weight reduction
  g. Ambulatory assists: canes, walkers
  h. Analgesics: aspirin (Ecotrin)
  i. NSAID: indomethacin (Indocin), ibuprofen (Motrin), sulindac (Clinoril), piroxicam (Feldene)
 7. Medical nursing interventions/responsibilities
  a. Maintain diet
  b. Assess musculoskeletal status
  c. Maintain joints in position of extension
  d. Monitor and record VS, UO, I/O
  e. Administer medications
  f. Encourage ventilation of feelings about change in body image
  g. Provide skin care
  h. Provide rest periods
  i. Assess ROM
  j. Maintain calorie count
  k. Assess pain
  l. Provide heat therapy: moist compresses, paraffin baths
  m. Teach body mechanics
  n. Provide passive ROM
 8. Patient/family teaching goals; the patient will:
  a. Keep follow-up appointments
  b. Maintain regular exercise program
  c. Maintain ideal weight
  d. State the action, side effects, and scheduling of medications
  e. Identify and reduce stress
  f. Recognize the signs and symptoms of skin breakdown
  g. Adhere to activity limitations
  h. Alternate rest periods with activity
  i. Follow dietary recommendations and restrictions
  j. Promote a safe environment
  k. Seek help from community agencies and resources

l.   Alter ADL to compensate for limited ROM
        m. Complete daily skin and foot care
        n. Use good body mechanics
    9. Possible medical complications: contractures
    10. Possible surgical interventions
        a. Synovectomy (see page 48)
        b. Arthrodesis (see page 48)
        c. Joint replacement (see page 48)

P. Gouty arthritis
    1. Definition: inflammatory joint disease caused by deposit of uric acid crystals
    2. Possible etiology
        a. Genetics
        b. Decreased uric acid excretion
        c. Chronic renal failure
        d. Myxedema
        e. Polycythemia vera
        f. Hyperparathyroidism
    3. Pathophysiology
        a. End product of purine metabolism is uric acid
        b. Abnormal purine metabolism results in decreased urinary secretion of
            urates and increased blood levels of uric acid
        c. Uric acid forms a precipitate in areas where blood flow is slowest
        d. Genetic defect in purine metabolism can lead to an overproduction of
            uric acid
    4. Possible clinical manifestations
        a. Joint pain
        b. Redness, swelling in joints
        c. Tophi: great toe, ankle, outer ear
        d. Malaise
        e. Tachycardia
        f. Elevated skin temperature
    5. Possible diagnostic test findings
        a. Hematology: increased ESR
        b. Blood chemistry: increased uric acid
        c. Synovial fluid analysis: sodium urate crystals
    6. Medical management
        a. Diet therapy: low-purine, alkaline-ash; force fluid intake to 3,000 ml/
            day; avoid shellfish, liver, sardines, anchovies, kidneys
        b. Activity: as tolerated
        c. Monitoring: VS, UO, I/O
        d. Laboratory studies: uric acid, ESR
        e. Exercise program
        f. Uricosuric agents: probenecid (Benemid), sulfinpyrazone (Anturane)
        g. Xanthine-oxidase inhibitors: allopurinal (Zyloprim)

      h. Antigout: colchicine (Colsalide)

      i. Analgesics: aspirin (Ecotrin)

      j. NSAID: indomethacin (Indocin), ibuprofen (Motrin), sulindac (Clinoril), piroxicam (Feldene)

7. Medical nursing interventions/responsibilities

      a. Maintain diet

      b. Force fluids to 3,000 ml/day

      c. Assess integumentary status

      d. Monitor and record VS, UO, I/O, laboratory studies

      e. Administer medications

      f. Allay anxiety

      g. Provide skin care

      h. Assess joints: pain, edema, ROM

      i. Provide bed cradle

      j. Reinforce exercise of joints

8. Patient/family teaching goals; the patient will:

      a. Keep follow-up appointments

      b. Maintain regular exercise program

      c. Maintain ideal weight

      d. State the action, side effects, and scheduling of medications

      e. Identify and reduce stress

      f. Recognize the signs and symptoms of gout

      g. Alternate rest periods with activity

      h. Follow dietary recommendations and restrictions

      i. Avoid fasting

      j. Limit alcohol intake

      k. Complete daily skin and foot care

9. Possible medical complications

      a. Renal calculi

      b. Cartilage damage

10. Possible surgical interventions: none

Q. Osteomyelitis

1. Definition: bone and soft-tissue bacterial infection

2. Possible etiology

      a. *Staphylococcus aureus*

      b. Hemolytic streptococcus

      c. Open trauma

      d. Infection

3. Pathophysiology

      a. Organism reaches bone through an open wound or via the bloodstream

      b. Infection causes bone destruction

      c. Bone fragments necrose (sequestra)

      d. New bone cells form over the sequestrum during healing process, resulting in nonunion

4. Possible clinical manifestations
   a. Malaise
   b. Elevated body temperature
   c. Bone pain
   d. Tachycardia
   e. Localized edema and redness
   f. Muscle spasms
   g. Increased pain with movement
5. Possible diagnostic test findings
   a. Blood cultures: positive identification of organism
   b. Hematology: increased WBC, ESR
   c. Wound culture: positive identification of organism
6. Medical management
   a. Diet therapy: high-calorie, high-vitamin C, high-protein
   b. I.V. therapy: heparin lock
   c. Activity: bed rest
   d. Monitoring: VS, UO, I/O, neurovascular checks
   e. Laboratory studies: WBC, ESR
   f. Nutritional support: I.V. hyperalimentation (IVH)
   g. Precautions: wound and skin
   h. Antibiotics: organism specific
   i. Analgesics: oxycodone HCl (Tylox)
   j. Continuous wound irrigation
   k. Heat therapy
   l. Cast or splint on affected body part
   m. Antipyretics: aspirin (Ecotrin)
7. Medical nursing interventions/responsibilities
   a. Maintain diet
   b. Force fluids to 3,000 ml/day
   c. Administer I.V. fluids
   d. Assess integumentary status
   e. Maintain patency of wound irrigation
   f. Monitor and record VS, UO, I/O, laboratory studies
   g. Administer IVH
   h. Administer medications
   i. Encourage ventilation of feelings about change in body image
   j. Provide skin care
   k. Turn every 2 hours
   l. Immobilize affected body part
   m. Maintain proper alignment
   n. Maintain bedrest
   o. Provide cast and splint care
   p. Assess pain
8. Patient/family teaching goals; the patient will:
   a. Keep follow-up appointments
   b. Maintain regular exercise program

      c. Maintain ideal weight
      d. State the action, side effects, and scheduling of medications
      e. Recognize the signs and symptoms of fractures
      f. Adhere to activity limitations
      g. Avoid exposure to people with infections
      h. Alternate rest periods with activity
      i. Monitor self for infection
      j. Follow dietary recommendations and restrictions
      k. Promote a safe environment
      l. Maintain a quiet environment
      m. Seek help from community agencies and resources
      n. Alter ADL to compensate for immobilization
      o. State health practices to avoid the spread of infection
      p. Avoid bearing weight on affected part
  9. Possible medical complications
      a. Bone necrosis
      b. Pathological fractures
      c. Sepsis
 10. Possible surgical interventions
      a. Incision and drainage of bone abscess
      b. Sequestrectomy

R. Osteoporosis
  1. Definition: metabolic bone dysfunction that results in reduced bone mass and increased porosity
  2. Possible etiology
      a. Lowered estrogen levels
      b. Immobility
      c. Liver disease
      d. Calcium deficiency
      e. Vitamin D deficiency
      f. Protein deficiency
      g. Bone marrow disorders
      h. Lack of exercise
      i. Increased phosphorus
      j. Cushing's syndrome
      k. Hyperthyroidism
  3. Pathophysiology
      a. Rate of bone resorption exceeds the rate of bone formation
      b. Increased phosphate stimulates parathyroid activity, which increases bone resorption
      c. Estrogens decrease bone resorption
  4. Possible clinical manifestations
      a. Dowager's hump (kyphosis)
      b. Back pain: thoracic and lumbar
      c. Loss of height

     d. Unsteady gait
     e. Joint pain
     f. Weakness
5. Possible diagnostic X-ray findings: thin, porous bone, increased vertebral curvature
6. Medical management
     a. Diet therapy: high-calcium, high-protein, high-vitamin and mineral
     b. Activity: as tolerated
     c. Monitoring: VS, UO, I/O
     d. Laboratory studies: calcium, phosphorus
     e. Estrogen: estradiol (Estrace)
     f. Calcium supplements: calcium carbonate (Os-Cal)
     g. Vitamin and mineral supplements
     h. Exercise program
7. Medical nursing interventions/responsibilities
     a. Maintain diet
     b. Assess musculoskeletal status
     c. Monitor and record VS, UO, I/O, laboratory studies
     d. Administer medications
     e. Encourage ventilation of feelings about change in body image
     f. Reinforce exercise program
     g. Teach good body mechanics and posture
     h. Assess pain
8. Patient/family teaching goals; the patient will:
     a. Keep follow-up appointments
     b. Maintain regular exercise program
     c. Maintain ideal weight
     d. State the action, side effects, and scheduling of medications
     e. Alternate rest periods with activity
     f. Follow dietary recommendations and restrictions
     g. Promote a safe environment
     h. Use good body mechanics
9. Possible medical complications: fractures
10. Possible surgical interventions: none

S. Osteogenic sarcoma (osteosarcoma)
1. Definition: malignant bone tumor that invades the ends of long bones
2. Possible etiology
     a. Osteoblastic activity
     b. Osteolytic activity
3. Pathophysiology
     a. Unregulated cell growth and uncontrolled cell division result in the development of a neoplasm
     b. Tumor arises from osteoblasts and dissolves the bone and soft tissue
     c. Metastasis may spread to the lung

4. Possible clinical manifestations
   a. Pain
   b. Limited movement
   c. Pathologic fractures
   d. Soft tissue mass over the tumor site
   e. Warm tissue over the tumor site
   f. Elevated body temperature
5. Possible diagnostic test findings
   a. Bone scan: presence of mass
   b. Biopsy: cytology positive for cancer cells
   c. Computerized tomography (CT) scan: presence of mass
   d. Blood chemistry: increased alkaline phosphatase
   e. Bone marrow aspiration: presence of cancer cells
6. Medical management
   a. Diet therapy: high-protein
   b. I.V. therapy: heparin lock
   c. Activity: as tolerated
   d. Monitoring: VS, UO, I/O
   e. Laboratory studies: calcium, phosphorus
   f. Antiemetics: prochlorperazine (Compazine)
   g. Nutritional support: IVH
   h. Radiation therapy
   i. Analgesics: oxycodone HCl (Tylox)
   j. Antineoplastics: cyclophosphamide (Cytoxan), vincristine sulfate (Oncovin)
   k. Chemotherapy
7. Medical nursing interventions/responsibilities
   a. Maintain diet
   b. Assess integumentary and musculoskeletal status
   c. Monitor and record VS, UO, I/O, laboratory studies
   d. Administer IVH
   e. Administer medications
   f. Encourage ventilation of feelings about change in body image and fear of dying
   g. Provide skin and mouth care
   h. Provide postchemotherapeutic and/or postradiation nursing care: provide skin, mouth, and perineal care; encourage dietary intake; administer antiemetics and antidiarrheals; monitor for bleeding, infection, and electrolyte imbalance; provide rest periods
   i. Assess pain
8. Patient/family teaching goals; the patient will:
   a. Keep follow-up appointments
   b. Maintain regular exercise program
   c. Maintain ideal weight

     d. State the action, side effects, and scheduling of medications
     e. Recognize the signs and symptoms of fracture
     f. Avoid exposure to people with infections
     g. Alternate rest periods with activity
     h. Monitor self for infection
     i. Follow dietary recommendations and restrictions
     j. Promote a safe environment
     k. Seek help from community agencies and resources
     l. Alter ADL to compensate for musculoskeletal deficits
     m. Complete daily skin care
     n. Use ambulation assists: crutches, cane, walker
  9. Possible medical complications
     a. Metastasis
     b. Pathologic fractures
 10. Possible surgical interventions: amputation (see page 50)

T. Carpal tunnel syndrome
  1. Definition: chronic compression neuropathy of the median nerve at the wrist
  2. Possible etiology
     a. Strenuous and repetitive use of the hands
     b. Fractures and dislocations of the wrist
     c. Bruising of the wrist
     d. Menopause
     e. Genetics
     f. Pregnancy
     g. Tenosynovitis
     h. Rheumatoid arthritis
     i. Acromegaly
     j. Hyperparathyroidism
     k. Obesity
     l. Gout
     m. Amyloidosis
  3. Pathophysiology
     a. Median nerve supplies sensory innervation to the palmar surface of the thumb and the first three fingers
     b. Median nerve also supplies motor innervation to the wrist and finger flexion
     c. Compression of the median nerve in the space between the inelastic transverse carpal ligament and the bones of the wrist (carpal tunnel) leads to pain and numbness in thumb, index, middle, and half of ring finger
  4. Possible clinical manifestations
     a. Nocturnal pain and paresthesia in thumb and first three fingers of the hand that is relieved by shaking the hands
     b. Burning and tingling of the hand
     c. Impaired sensation in the hand

    d. Pain radiating to forearm, shoulder, neck, and chest
    e. Thenar atrophy
    f. Loss of fine motor movement of the hand
5. Possible diagnostic test findings
    a. Tinel's sign: positive
    b. Phalen's sign: positive
    c. Motor nerve velocity studies: segmental, distal, median, and motor conduction delay, and conduction block at wrist
6. Medical management
    a. Diet therapy: low-sodium, restrict fluids
    b. Position: avoid flexion of wrist, elevate the hand
    c. Activity: avoid use of hand
    d. Monitoring: VS, UO, I/O, neurovascular checks
    e. Treatment: hand splint
    f. Analgesics: acetaminophen (Tylenol)
    g. Diuretics: furosemide (Lasix)
    h. Glucocorticoids: cortisone (Cortone)
7. Medical nursing interventions/responsibilities
    a. Maintain diet
    b. Assess neurovascular status
    c. Elevate hand
    d. Monitor and record VS
    e. Administer medications
    f. Encourage ventilation of feelings about inability to use hand and perform job requirements
    g. Provide skin care
    h. Provide ROM to splinted hand
    i. Protect hand from cold, local trauma, burns, abrasions, and chemical irritations
    j. Avoid manual activity that includes dorsiflexion and volar flexion of wrist
8. Patient/family teaching goals; the patient will:
    a. Keep follow-up appointments
    b. Maintain ROM exercise program for the hand
    c. Maintain ideal weight
    d. State the action, side effects, and scheduling of medications
    e. Identify and reduce activities that increase pain
    f. Recognize the signs and symptoms of skin breakdown and contracture
    g. Adhere to activity limitations
    h. Alternate rest periods with activities involving the hand
    i. Follow dietary recommendations and restrictions
    j. Alter ADL to compensate for neuromuscular deficits
    k. Complete daily skin care
    l. Protect hand from trauma
    m. Splint hand
    n. Evaluate need for vocational retraining

9. Possible medical complications
   a. Contracture
   b. "Ape hand" (loss of thumb abduction and opposition)
   c. Trophic changes of tips of thumbs, index and middle fingers
10. Possible surgical interventions: carpal tunnel release (see page 51)

U. Herniated nucleus pulposa (HNP, "slipped disc")

1. Definition
   a. Rupture of intervertebral disc
   b. Types: lumbrosacral (L4, L5); cervical (C5, C6, C7)
2. Possible etiology
   a. Accidents
   b. Back or neck strain
   c. Congenital bone deformity
   d. Degeneration of disc
   e. Weakness of ligaments
   f. Heavy lifting
   g. Trauma
3. Pathophysiology
   a. Protrusion of the nucleus pulposa into the spinal canal compresses the spinal cord or nerve roots
   b. Compression of the spinal cord or nerve roots causes pain, numbness, and loss of motor function
4. Possible clinical manifestations
   a. Acute pain in lower back radiating across buttock and down leg
   b. Weakness, numbness, and tingling of foot and leg or hand
   c. Neck stiffness
   d. Neck pain that radiates down the arm to the hand
   e. Weakness of affected upper extremities
   f. Atrophy of biceps and triceps
   g. Straightening of normal lumbar curve with scoliosis away from affected side
   h. Pain on ambulation
5. Possible diagnostic test findings
   a. Lasegue's sign: positive
   b. CSF analysis: increased protein
   c. Myelogram: compression of spinal cord
   d. Electromyography (EMG): presence of spinal nerve involvement
   e. X-ray: narrowing of disc space
   f. Tendon reflexes: depressed or absent Achilles reflex
6. Medical management
   a. Diet therapy: calories according to metabolic needs, high-roughage; force fluids
   b. Position: semi-Fowler
   c. Activity: bed rest, active and passive ROM, isometric exercises

    d. Monitoring: VS, UO, I/O, neurovascular checks, laboratory studies
    e. Treatments: heating pad; moist, hot compresses
    f. Orthopedic devices: back brace, cervical collar
    g. Analgesics: oxycodone hydrochloride (Tylox)
    h. Antacids: magnesium and aluminum hydroxide (Maalox), aluminum hydroxide gel (Gelusil)
    i. Sedatives: phenobarbital (Luminal)
    j. Stool softeners: docusate sodium (Colace)
    k. Pelvic traction
    l. Cervical traction
    m. Muscle relaxants: diazepam (Valium)
    n. Chemonucleolysis using chymopapain (Discase)
    o. NSAID: indomethacin (Indocin), ibuprofen (Motrin), sulindac (Clinoril), piroxicam (Feldene)
    p. Corticosteroids: cortisone (Cortone)

7. Medical nursing interventions/responsibilities
    a. Maintain diet with increased fluids
    b. Assess neurovascular status
    c. Maintain semi-Fowler position with moderate hip and knee flexion
    d. Monitor and record VS, UO, I/O, laboratory studies
    e. Administer medications
    f. Encourage ventilation of feelings about change in body image, fears about present and future disability
    g. Provide skin and back care
    h. Turn every 2 hours using logrolling technique
    i. Maintain bed rest and body alignment
    j. Maintain traction, braces, and/or cervical collar
    k. Promote independence in ADL
    l. Apply bedboards

8. Patient/family teaching goals; the patient will:
    a. Keep follow-up appointments
    b. Maintain regular exercise program and muscle strengthening and stretching exercises
    c. Maintain ideal weight
    d. State the action, side effects, and scheduling of medications
    e. Recognize the signs and symptoms of neuromuscular deficits
    f. Adhere to activity limitations: avoid lifting, climbing stairs, riding in car, sleeping prone
    g. Alternate rest periods with activity
    h. Follow dietary recommendations and restrictions
    i. Alter ADL to compensate for neuromuscular deficits
    j. Use proper body mechanics and maintain posture
    k. Avoid flexion, extension, and rotation of neck
    l. Use a single pillow
    m. Use orthopedic assistive devices

9. Possible medical complications
    a. Upper respiratory infection
    b. Urinary tract infection
    c. Thrombophlebitis
    d. Chronic pain
    e. Muscle atrophy
    f. Progressive paralysis
10. Possible surgical interventions
    a. Laminectomy (see page 54)
    b. Spinal fusion (see page 55)

V. Fractures

1. Definition
    a. Break in the continuity of bone
    b. Types: complete, incomplete, comminuted, greenstick, simple, compound, transverse, spiral, oblique, depressed, compression, avulsion, and pathologic
    c. Types of fractured hip: intracapsular, extracapsular, or intertrochanteric
2. Possible etiology
    a. Trauma
    b. Osteoporosis
    c. Multiple myeloma
    d. Bone tumors
    e. Immobility
    f. Malnutrition
    g. Cushing's syndrome
    h. Osteomyelitis
    i. Steroid therapy
    j. Aging process
3. Pathophysiology
    a. Fracture occurs when the stress placed on the bone is more than the bone can absorb
    b. Localized tissue injury results in muscle spasm, edema, hemorrhage, compressed nerves, and ecchymosis
4. Possible clinical manifestations
    a. Pain aggravated by motion
    b. Tenderness over fracture site
    c. Loss of function or motion
    d. Edema
    e. Crepitus
    f. Ecchymosis
    g. Deformity
    h. False motion
    i. Paresthesia
    j. Affected leg appears shorter (fractured hip)

5. Possible diagnostic test findings
   a. X-ray: break in continuity of bone
   b. Hematology: decreased Hgb and Hct
6. Medical management
   a. Diet therapy: high-protein, high-vitamin, low-calcium; increased fluid intake
   b. Position: elevate affected extremity (fractures); flat with leg in abducted position (fractured hip)
   c. Activity: as tolerated (fractures); active and passive ROM on unaffected limbs (fractured hip); isometric exercises
   d. Monitoring: VS, UO, I/O, neurovascular checks
   e. Laboratory studies: Hgb, Hct, phosphorus, calcium
   f. Treatments: cast care, pin care, ice packs, incentive spirometry, abductor pillow (fractured hip)
   g. Analgesics: oxycodone hydrochloride (Tylox)
   h. Skin traction: Buck's, Bryant's, or Russell's
   i. Skeletal traction: Thomas splint with Pearson attachment, Steinmann pin, Kirchner wire, or Crutchfield tongs
   j. Closed reduction with hip spica cast (fractured hip)
   k. Cast or closed reduction (fracture)
7. Medical nursing interventions/responsibilities
   a. Maintain diet with increased fluid
   b. Assess neurovascular and respiratory status
   c. Maintain flat position with foot of bed elevated 25° (fractured hip)
   d. Maintain legs in abduction (fractured hip)
   e. Maintain elevation of affected extremity (fracture)
   f. Monitor and record VS, UO, I/O, laboratory studies
   g. Administer medications
   h. Allay anxiety
   i. Provide skin, pin, and cast care
   j. Turn every 2 hours to unaffected side using logrolling technique (fractured hip)
   k. Maintain extended position of hip (fractured hip)
   l. Maintain activity as tolerated (fractures)
   m. Promote independence in ADL
   n. Provide active and passive ROM and isometric exercises on unaffected limbs
   o. Provide trapeze
   p. Maintain traction
   q. Keep side rails up
   r. Provide appropriate sensory stimulation with frequent reorientation
   s. Provide pulmonary toilet: TCDB, incentive spirometry
   t. Provide cast care
   u. Prevent constipation

      v. Maintain proper body alignment
      w. Assess pin sites for infection
      x. Provide diversional activity
      y. Provide heel and elbow protectors and sheepskin
      z. Apply antiembolitic stockings

8. Patient/family teaching goals; the patient will:
   a. Keep follow-up appointments
   b. State the action, side effects, and scheduling of medications
   c. Recognize the signs and symptoms of decreased circulation and infection
   d. Adhere to activity limitations
   e. Alternate rest periods with activity
   f. Follow dietary recommendations and restrictions
   g. Promote a safe environment
   h. Alter ADL to compensate for altered mobility and neuromuscular function
   i. Complete daily skin and foot care
   j. Demonstrate use of ambulation assists in ADL
   k. Demonstrate cast care (fracture)
   l. Maintain regular exercise program with ROM and iosmetric exercises
   m. Maintain ideal weight

9. Possible medical complications
   a. Deep vein thrombosis
   b. Anemia
   c. Fat embolism
   d. Pulmonary embolism
   e. Renal lithiasis
   f. Pneumonia
   g. Urinary tract infections
   h. Compartmental syndrome (fracture)
   i. Hypovolemic shock
   j. Nonunion
   k. Osteomyelitis (fracture)
   l. Avascular necrosis of the femoral head (fractured hip)
   m. Decubiti

10. Possible surgical interventions
    a. ORIF (see page 53)
    b. External fixation (fractures) (see page 49)

W. Systemic lupus erythematosus (SLE)

1. Definition: chronic connective tissue disease involving multiple organ systems
2. Possible etiology
   a. Unknown
   b. Genetic

    c. Autoimmune disease

    d. Viral

    e. Drug-induced: procainamide (Pronestyl) and hydralazine (Apresoline)

3. Pathophysiology

    a. Defect in body's immunologic mechanism produces serum auto-antibodies directed against components of patient's own cell nuclei

    b. Deposits of antigen/antibody complexes affect connective cells throughout the body, including blood vessels, mucous membranes, joints, skin, kidneys, muscles, brain, and heart

4. Possible clinical manifestations

    a. Oral and nasopharyngeal ulcerations

    b. Alopecia

    c. Photosensitivity

    d. Early morning joint stiffness

    e. Low-grade fever

    f. Butterfly erythema on face

    g. Erythema on palms

    h. Muscle pain

    i. Abdominal pain

    j. Malaise and weakness

    k. Weight loss

    l. Lymphadenopathy

    m. Anorexia

5. Possible diagnostic test findings

    a. Hematology: decreased Hgb, Hct, WBC, platelets; increased ESR

    b. Rheumatoid factor: positive

    c. LE prep: positive

    d. Urine chemistry: proteinuria, hematuria

    e. Blood chemistry: decreased complement fixation

    f. ANA test: positive

6. Medical management

    a. Diet therapy: high-iron, high-protein, high vitamins, especially vitamin C

    b. I.V. therapy: heparin lock

    c. Activity: as tolerated

    d. Monitoring: VS, UO, I/O

    e. Laboratory studies: Hgb, Hct, WBC, platelets, ESR, BUN, Cr

    f. Plasmapheresis

    g. Precautions: seizure

    h. Analgesics: acetaminophen (Tylenol)

    i. Antacids: magnesium and aluminum hydroxide (Maalox), aluminum hydroxide gel (Gelusil)

    j. Corticosteroids: prednisone (Deltasone)

    k. Antimalarials: hydroxychloroquine (Plaquenil)

    l. Antipyretics: aspirin (Ecotrin)

     m. NSAID: indomethacin (Indocin), ibuprofen (Motrin)

     n. Hematinics: ferrous sulfate (Feosol), ferrous gluconate (Fergon)

     o. Immunosuppressive agents: azathioprine (Imuran), cyclophosphamide (Cytoxan)

     p. Vitamins and minerals

7. Medical nursing interventions/responsibilities
   a. Maintain diet
   b. Assess musculoskeletal and renal status
   c. Monitor and record VS, UO, I/O, laboratory studies, daily weights
   d. Administer medications
   e. Encourage ventilation of feelings about change in body image and chronic nature of disease
   f. Provide skin and mouth care
   g. Avoid exposure to sunlight
   h. Minimize environmental stress
   i. Maintain seizure precautions
   j. Provide rest periods
   k. Prevent infection
   l. Maintain a quiet environment
   m. Avoid use of dusting powder
   n. Promote independence in ADL
   o. Provide postchemotherapeutic and/or postradiation nursing care: provide skin, mouth, and perineal care; encourage dietary intake; administer antiemetics and antidiarrheals; monitor for bleeding, infection, and electrolyte imbalance

8. Patient/family teaching goals; the patient will:
   a. Keep follow-up appointments
   b. Maintain regular exercise program
   c. Stop smoking
   d. Maintain ideal weight
   e. State the action, side effects, and scheduling of medications
   f. Identify and reduce stress
   g. Recognize the signs and symptoms of renal failure
   h. Avoid exposure to people with infections
   i. Alternate rest periods with activity
   j. Monitor self for infection
   k. Follow dietary recommendations and restrictions
   l. Maintain a quiet environment
   m. Seek help from community agencies and resources
   n. Alter ADL to compensate for fatigue and joint pain
   o. Complete daily skin and mouth care
   p. Avoid over-the-counter medications
   q. Avoid exposure to sunlight and use of hair spray, hair coloring, and oral contraceptives

    r. Use liquid cosmetics to cover rashes

    s. Reinforce independence in ADL

9. Possible medication complications

    a. Necrosis of glomerular capillaries

    b. Inflammation of cerebral and ocular blood vessels

    c. Necrosis of lymph nodes

    d. Vasculitis of gastrointestinal tract and pleura

    e. Degeneration of basal layer of the skin

    f. Congestive heart failure (CHF)

    g. Seizures

    h. Depression

    i. Infection

    j. Peripheral neuropathy

10. Possible surgical interventions: none

Points to Remember

Metabolic illnesses or medications that cause osteoporosis increase the risk of skeletal fracture.

Alterations in mobility that result from musculoskeletal disorders affect a patient's occupational, recreational, and social activities.

Range-of-motion activities and proper alignment reduce the occurrence of contractures.

Pain control is a primary focus for the nursing management of patients with musculoskeletal disorders.

Nursing assessment of the patient with musculoskeletal disorders should include monitoring for complications of immobility.

Glossary

Crepitation — grating sound produced by bone rubbing against bone.

Pannus — granular tissue that covers and invades articular cartilage.

Subluxation — partial dislocation of a joint.

Thenar — musculature at base of thumb.

Tophi — urate crystals which are deposited in areas of diminished blood flow, such as joints and ear lobes.

Nervous System

Learning Objectives

After studying this section, the reader should be able to:

- Describe the psychosocial impact of nervous system disorders.

- Differentiate between modifiable and nonmodifiable risk factors in the development of a nervous system disorder.

- List three potential and three actual nursing diagnoses for the patient with a nervous system disorder.

- Identify the medical and surgical nursing interventions/responsibilities for the patient with a nervous system disorder.

- Write three teaching goals for the patient with a nervous system disorder.

III. Nervous System

A. Anatomy and physiology

1. Neuron
   a. Nerve cell, or neuron, is the basic functional unit of the nervous system
   b. It is composed of a cell body, dendrite, and axon, surrounded by a myelin sheath
   c. It conducts impulses across a synapse to muscles, glands, and organs in the central nervous system
   d. Neurotransmitters (acetylcholine and norepinephrine) help conduct impulses across the synapse
2. Central nervous system (CNS)
   a. The CNS includes the brain and spinal cord
   b. Nervous system has two divisions: CNS and peripheral nervous system (PNS)
   c. Meninges are protective membranous layers that cover and protect CNS
   d. Meninges are composed of dura mater, pia mater, and arachnoid membrane
   e. Four ventricles produce and circulate cerebrospinal fluid (CSF)
   f. CSF surrounds and protects brain and spinal cord
   g. CSF exchanges nutrients and wastes at the cellular level
3. Brain
   a. Structure: cerebrum, diencephalon, brain stem, and cerebellum
   b. Cerebrum: divided into two hemispheres that contain four lobes each
   c. Frontal lobe: site of personality, intellectual functioning, and motor speech
   d. Parietal lobe: site of sensation, integration of sensory information, spatial relationships
   e. Temporal lobe: site of hearing, taste, smell, and sensory speech
   f. Occipital lobe: site of vision
   g. Blood supply to brain: internal carotid arteries, vertebral arteries, circle of Willis
   h. Diencephalon: composed of thalamus and hypothalamus
   i. Thalamus: relays sensory impulses of pain, temperature, and touch to the cortex
   j. Hypothalamus: controls temperature, respiration, blood pressure, and emotional states
   k. Brain stem: composed of midbrain, pons, and medulla oblongata
   l. Medulla oblongata: contains vomiting, vasomotor, respiratory, and cardiac centers
   m. Pyramidal tracts: decussate at the medulla oblongata
   n. Cerebellum: coordinates muscle tone and movement, equilibrium and posture
4. Spinal cord
   a. It is composed of grey matter and white matter
   b. Grey matter forms H-shaped core in the spinal cord

    c. White matter includes the ascending tracts (sensory) and descending tracts (motor) of the spinal cord

    d. Reflex arc is the involuntary response to a stimulus

5. Peripheral nervous system (PNS)

    a. Structure: 12 pairs of cranial nerves, 31 pairs of spinal nerves, and the autonomic nervous system

    b. Cranial nerves: olfactory, optic, oculomotor, trochlear, trigeminal, abducens, facial, acoustic, glossopharyngeal, vagus, accessory, and hypoglossal nerves

    c. Spinal nerves: carry mixed impulses (motor and sensory) to and from the spinal cord

    d. Autonomic nervous system: composed of sympathetic nervous system (SNS) and parasympathetic nervous system; regulates smooth muscle, cardiac muscle, and glands

    e. SNS activity: results in adrenergic responses

    f. Parasympathetic activity: results in cholinergic responses

B. Physical assessment findings

1. Subjective data that often accompany nervous system disorders

    a. Memory impairment

    b. Numbness and tingling

    c. Muscle weakness

    d. Twitching and spasm

    e. Ringing in ears

    f. Difficulty chewing, swallowing, talking, and walking

    g. Headache

    h. Dizziness

    i. Fainting

    j. Loss of balance and coordination

    k. Nausea and vomiting

    l. Pain

    m. Mental confusion or excitement

    n. Blurred or double vision

    o. Change in bowel and bladder patterns

    p. Sexual dysfunction

    q. Tremors

    r. Stiff neck

    s. Drooping eyelids

2. Objective data to evaluate in nervous system disorders

    a. Paresthesia

    b. Change in level of consciousness

    c. Ataxic gait

    d. Dyskinesia

    e. Tinnitus

    f. Dysphagia
    g. Aphasia
    h. Seizures
    i. Diplopia
    j. Papilledema
    k. Change in visual fields
    l. Loss of vision
    m. Temperature
    n. Pulse changes
    o. Character and pattern of respirations
    p. Hypertension
    q. Change in muscle reflexes
    r. Pupil size and reaction
    s. Positive Babinski reflex
    t. Loss of reflexes: cough, gag, corneal, oculocephalic and oculovestibular
    u. Ptosis

C. Diagnostic tests and procedures used to evaluate nervous system disorders
    1. Electroencephalography (EEG)
        a. Definition/purpose: noninvasive test that graphically represents the brain's electrical activity
        b. Nursing interventions/responsibilities: before procedure, assess patient's ability to lie still; reassure him that electrical shock will not occur; tell him that he may be subjected to various stimuli such as lights and sounds; hold medications and foods with caffeine
    2. Computerized tomography (CT)
        a. Definition/purpose: noninvasive scan that may use I.V. injection of contrast dye to visualize the brain and its structures
        b. Nursing interventions/responsibilities: before procedure, assess allergies to iodine, seafood, and radiopaque dyes; allay anxiety; inform patient he may feel flushing of the face and throat irritation
    3. Magnetic resonance imaging (MRI)
        a. Definition/purpose: noninvasive scan using magnetic and radio waves to visualize the brain and its structures
        b. Nursing interventions/responsibilities: before procedure, remove jewelry and metal objects from the patient; assess patient's ability to lie still; administer sedation as ordered. Caution: patients with pacemakers, surgical and orthopedic clips, or shrapnel cannot be scanned.
    4. Cerebral angiogram
        a. Definition/purpose: fluoroscopic examination of the cerebral arteries after injection of a radiopaque dye through a catheter
        b. Nursing interventions/responsibilities: before procedure, assess allergies to iodine, seafood, or radiopaque dyes; inform patient that he may feel flushing of face and throat irritation; after procedure, monitor vital signs (VS); allay anxiety; assess insertion site for bleeding; monitor neurovital signs

5. CSF analysis
   a. Definition/purpose: microscopic examination of CSF for blood, white blood cells (WBC), bacteria, protein, glucose, and electrolytes
   b. Nursing interventions/responsibilities: label and send specimens to the laboratory immediately
6. Lumbar puncture (LP)
   a. Definition/purpose: invasive procedure to collect CSF from the lumbar subarachnoid space and measure CSF pressure
   b. Nursing interventions/responsibilities: before procedure, assess patient's ability to lie still in flexed, lateral, recumbent position; after procedure, maintain flat bed rest for 24 hours; administer analgesics as ordered; assess puncture site for bleeding; monitor neurovital signs; force fluids
7. Electromyography (EMG)
   a. Definition/purpose: noninvasive test that graphically records the electrical activity of the muscle at rest and during contraction
   b. Nursing interventions/responsibilities: before procedure, advise the patient that he will be asked to flex and relax muscles during the procedure; after procedure, administer analgesics as ordered
8. Myelogram
   a. Definition/purpose: injection of radiopaque dye by lumbar puncture to visualize the subarachnoid space, spinal cord, and vertebral bodies under fluoroscopy
   b. Nursing interventions/responsibilities: before procedure, assess allergies to iodine, seafood, and radiopaque dyes; inform patient that he may feel flushing of the face and throat irritation; after procedure, maintain flat bed rest as ordered; assess insertion site for bleeding; monitor neurovital signs; force fluids
9. Brain scan
   a. Definition/purpose: visual imaging of blood flow distribution and structures of the brain after injection of a radiopaque dye
   b. Nursing interventions/responsibilities: before procedure, assess allergies to iodine, seafood, and radiopaque dyes; inform patient that he may feel flushing of the face and throat irritation; assess patient's ability to lie still during the procedure
10. Skull films
   a. Definition/purpose: radiographic picture of the bones of the head and neck
   b. Nursing interventions/responsibilities: before procedure, assess patient's ability to lie still during the procedure
11. Positron emission tomography (PET)
   a. Definition/purpose: visual imaging of oxygen uptake, blood flow, and glucose using injection of radioisotope
   b. Nursing interventions/responsibilities: before procedure, assess patient's ability to lie still during the procedure; withhold alcohol, tobacco, and caffeine 24 hours before procedure; hold medications as ordered; after procedure, assess insertion site

12. Blood chemistry
   a. Definition/purpose: laboratory analysis of blood sample for potassium, sodium, calcium, phosphorus, protein, albumin, osmolality, glucose, bicarbonate, BUN, and Cr
   b. Nursing interventions/responsibilities: before procedure, withhold food and fluids as ordered; after procedure, monitor site for bleeding
13. Hematologic studies
   a. Definition/purpose: laboratory analysis of blood sample for WBC, red blood cells (RBC), erythrocyte sedimentation rate (ESR), prothrombin time (PT), partial thromboplastin time (PTT), platelets, hemoglobin (Hgb), and hematocrit (Hct)
   b. Nursing interventions/responsibilities: assess site for bleeding; note current drug therapy

D. **Possible psychosocial impact of nervous system disorders**
   1. Developmental impact
      a. Change in body image
      b. Feelings of lack of control over body functions
      c. Fear of rejection
      d. Embarrassment from change in body structure and function
      e. Decreased self-esteem
      f. Fear of dying
      g. Dependency
   2. Economic impact
      a. Disruption or loss of employment
      b. Cost of hospitalizations
      c. Cost of home health care
      d. Cost of special equipment
   3. Occupational and recreational impact
      a. Restrictions in work activity
      b. Change in leisure activity
      c. Restrictions in physical activity
      d. Need for vocational retraining
   4. Social impact
      a. Change in eating modes
      b. Change in elimination patterns and modes
      c. Social isolation
      d. Change in sexual function
      e. Change in role performance

E. **Possible risk factors for development of nervous system disorders**
   1. Modifiable risk factors
      a. Exposure to chemical and environmental pollutants
      b. Substance abuse
      c. Participation in contact sports
      d. Hypertension

2. Nonmodifiable risk factors
   a. Aging process
   b. Family history of neurologic disease
   c. History of cardiac disease
   d. History of head injury
   e. Exposure to viral and bacterial infection

F. Possible nursing diagnoses for the patient with nervous system disorders
   1. Actual nursing diagnoses
      a. Impaired physical mobility
      b. Self-care deficit: feeding
      c. Self-care deficit: bathing
      d. Self-care deficit: hygiene
      e. Self-care deficit: dressing
      f. Self-care deficit: grooming
      g. Self-care deficit: toileting
      h. Sensory-perceptual alteration: visual
      i. Sensory-perceptual alteration: tactile
      j. Alteration in thought processes
      k. Social isolation
      l. Impaired home maintenance management
   2. Potential nursing diagnoses
      a. Sexual dysfunction
      b. Alteration in urinary elimination
      c. Impaired communication
      d. Alteration in bowel elimination: incontinence
      e. Alteration in nutrition: less than body requirements
      f. Ineffective airway clearance
      g. Ineffective individual coping
      h. Potential for injury
      i. Alteration in tissue perfusion: cerebral
      j. Powerlessness
      k. Potential for violence

G. Surgical intervention: craniotomy
   1. Definition
      a. Surgical opening in the skull to excise a tumor, evacuate a blood clot, relieve intracranial pressure, or clip an aneurysm
      b. Classified into supratentorial and infratentorial
   2. Preoperative surgical nursing interventions/responsibilities
      a. Complete patient and family preoperative teaching: assess understanding of surgical procedure; explain operating room (OR), recovery room (RR), preoperative and postoperative routine; demonstrate postoperative turning, coughing, and deep breathing (TCDB), splinting, leg exercises, and range-of-motion (ROM) exercises; explain postoperative need for

       drainage tubes, surgical dressings, oxygen therapy, I.V. therapy, and pain control

   b. Complete preoperative check list
   c. Administer preoperative medications
   d. Allay patient and family anxiety about surgery
   e. Document patient history and physical assessment data base
   f. Administer antibiotics
   g. Prepare the patient for preoperative shaving of the head

3. Postoperative surgical nursing interventions/responsibilities
   a. Assess cardiac, respiratory, and neurologic status
   b. Assess pain and administer postoperative analgesic
   c. Progress diet as tolerated
   d. Administer I.V. fluids and I.V. hyperalimentation (IVH)
   e. Allay anxiety
   f. Assess surgical dressing and change as directed
   g. Reinforce TCDB
   h. Maintain semi-Fowler position
   i. Assess for return of peristalsis
   j. Provide pulmonary toilet: incentive spirometry
   k. Maintain activity: as tolerated or passive ROM
   l. Administer oxygen and maintain endotracheal tube (ET) to ventilator
   m. Monitor VS, urinary output (UO), intake and output (I/O), central venous presure (CVP), laboratory studies, EKG, neurovital signs, neurovascular checks, intracranial pressure (ICP)
   n. Monitor and maintain position and patency of drainage tubes: nasogastric (NG), Foley, wound drainage
   o. Assess cough and gag reflex
   p. Encourage ventilation of feelings about change in body image, fear of dying
   q. Assess for signs of diabetes insipidus
   r. Provide eye care
   s. Allow a rest period between each nursing activity
   t. Assess for signs of increasing ICP
   u. Administer corticosteroids
   v. Administer anticonvulsants
   w. Administer laxatives
   x. Administer antacids
   y. Maintain seizure precautions

4. Possible surgical complications
   a. Increased ICP
   b. Seizures
   c. Respiratory distress
   d. Diabetes insipidus
   e. Motor and sensory deficits
   f. Infection
   g. Meningitis

5. Patient/family postoperative teaching goals; the patient will:
   a. Keep follow-up appointments
   b. Maintain regular exercise program
   c. Stop smoking
   d. Maintain ideal weight
   e. State the action, side effects, and scheduling of medications
   f. Recognize the signs and symptoms of infection, change in level of consciousness, seizure activity
   g. Adhere to activity limitations
   h. Complete daily incision care
   i. Provide a safe environment
   j. Seek help from community agencies and resources

H. Surgical intervention: endarterectomy
1. Definition: surgical removal of atheromas from arteries with a patch graft repair of the vessel
2. Preoperative surgical nursing interventions/responsibilities
   a. Complete patient and family preoperative teaching: assess understanding of surgical procedure; explain OR, RR, preoperative and postoperative routine; demonstrate postoperative TCDB, splinting, leg exercises, and ROM; explain postoperative need for drainage tubes, surgical dressings, oxygen therapy, I.V. therapy, and pain control
   b. Complete preoperative check list
   c. Administer preoperative medications
   d. Allay patient and family anxiety about surgery
   e. Document patient history and physical assessment data base
   f. Administer antibiotics
   g. Protect site from trauma
   h. Obtain preoperative vascular assessment
3. Postoperative surgical nursing interventions/responsibilities
   a. Assess cardiac, respiratory, and neurologic status
   b. Assess pain and administer postoperative analgesic
   c. Progress diet as tolerated
   d. Administer I.V. fluids
   e. Allay anxiety
   f. Assess surgical dressing and change as directed
   g. Reinforce TCDB
   h. Maintain semi-Fowler position
   i. Assess for return of peristalsis
   j. Provide pulmonary toilet: incentive spirometry
   k. Maintain activity: as tolerated, active/passive ROM, isometric exercises
   l. Administer oxygen
   m. Monitor VS, UO, I/O, laboratory studies, neurovital signs, neurovascular checks
   n. Monitor and maintain position and patency of drainage tubes: NG, Foley, wound drainage

       o. Assess site for bleeding
       p. Maintain pressure dressing
       q. Assess neck edema for carotid endarterectomy
       r. Assess ability to swallow for carotid endarterectomy
  4. Possible surgical complications
       a. Bleeding
       b. Embolus
       c. Thrombus
       d. Neurological deficits
       e. Infection
  5. Patient/family postoperative teaching goals; the patient will:
       a. Keep follow-up appointments
       b. Maintain regular exercise program
       c. Stop smoking
       d. Maintain ideal weight
       e. State the action, side effects, and scheduling of medications
       f. Recognize the signs and symptoms of infection, motor and sensory deficits
       g. Adhere to activity limitations
       h. Complete daily incision care

I. Parkinson's disease (paralysis agitans)
  1. Definition: progressive degenerative disease of the extrapyramidal system associated with dopamine deficiency
  2. Possible etiology
       a. Neuromuscular imbalance of dopamine and acetylcholine
       b. Cerebral vascular disease
       c. Drug-induced: phentolamine (reserpine), methlydopa (Aldomet)
       d. Dopamine deficiency
       e. Unknown
  3. Pathophysiology
       a. Nerve cells in basal ganglia are destroyed, resulting in decreased muscular function
       b. Dopamine in the substantia nigra degenerates
       c. Lack of dopamine results in loss of inhibitory synaptic transmitter for muscle tone and coordination
  4. Possible clinical manifestations
       a. "Pill rolling" tremors
       b. Shuffling gait
       c. Stiff joints
       d. Masklike facial expression
       e. Dyskinesia
       f. Dysphagia
       g. Drooling

    h. Cogwheel rigidity
    i. Fatigue
    j. Stooped posture
    k. Tremors at rest
    l. Small handwriting
5. Possible diagnostic test findings
    a. EEG: minimal slowing
    b. CT scan: normal
6. Medical management
    a. Diet therapy: high-residue, high-calorie, soft
    b. Physical therapy
    c. Activity: as tolerated
    d. Monitoring: VS, UO, I/O, neurovital signs
    e. Anticholinergics: benztropine mesylate (Cogentin), trihexyphenidyl (Artane)
    f. Antiparkinsonian agents: levodopa (L-Dopa), Carbidopa (Sinemet), benztropine mesylate (Cogentin)
    g. Antispasmodics: procyclidine HCl (Kemadrin)
    h. Antidepressants: amitriptyline HCl (Elavil)
    i. Antiviral: amantadine (Symmetrel)
7. Medical nursing interventions/responsibilities
    a. Maintain diet
    b. Assess neurovascular and respiratory status
    c. Position patient to prevent contractures
    d. Monitor and record VS, UO, I/O
    e. Administer medications
    f. Encourage ventilation of feelings about change in body image
    g. Ambulate patient daily
    h. Maintain airway
    i. Provide active and passive ROM
    j. Provide daily skin care
    k. Provide oral hygiene
    l. Reinforce gait training
    m. Reinforce independence in care
8. Patient/family postoperative teaching goals; the patient will:
    a. Keep follow-up appointments
    b. Maintain regular exercise program
    c. State the action, side effects, and scheduling of medications
    d. Recognize the signs and symptoms of respiratory distress
    e. Alternate rest periods with activity
    f. Promote a safe environment
    g. Seek help from community agencies and resources
    h. Use measures to prevent choking: cut food into small pieces, suction mouth frequently, soft diet

       i. Avoid food high in vitamin B_6: tuna, pork, dried beans, salmon, beef liver

       j. Increase intake of roughage and fluids to prevent constipation

  9. Possible medical complications

     a. Depression

     b. Corneal ulceration

     c. Injury

     d. Aspiration

     e. Constipation

10. Possible surgical interventions: stereotaxic thalamotomy to relieve tremor and rigidity

J. Multiple sclerosis

  1. Definition: progressive disease of impaired motor nerve conduction

  2. Possible etiology

     a. Unknown

     b. Autoimmune disease

     c. Viral

  3. Pathophysiology

     a. Scattered demyelinization occurs in the brain and spinal cord

     b. Degeneration of myelin sheath results in patches of sclerotic tissue and impaired conduction of motor nerve impulses

  4. Possible clinical manifestations

     a. Weakness

     b. Nystagmus

     c. Scanning speech

     d. Ataxia

     e. Diplopia

     f. Paresthesia

     g. Blurred vision

     h. Impaired sensation

     i. Feelings of euphoria

     j. Paralysis

     k. Urinary incontinence

     l. Intention tremor

     m. Loss of position sense

  5. Possible diagnostic test findings

     a. CSF analysis: increased IgG, protein, WBC

     b. CT scan: normal except in chronic illness, when atrophy is found

     c. MRI: normal except in chronic illness, when atrophy is found

  6. Medical management

     a. Diet therapy: high-calorie, high-protein, high-vitamin, gluten-free

     b. Activity: as tolerated

     c. Monitoring: VS, UO, I/O, neurovital signs

     d. Speech therapy

     e. Plasmapheresis

    f. Muscle relaxants: baclofen (Lioresal)
    g. Physical therapy
    h. Glucocorticoids: prednisone (Deltasone), dexamethasone (Decadron), corticotropin (ACTH)
    i. Antacids: magnesium and aluminum hydroxide (Maalox), aluminum hydroxide gel (Alternagel)
    j. Fluids: force intake

7. Medical nursing interventions/responsibilities
    a. Maintain diet
    b. Force fluids
    c. Assess neurologic status
    d. Monitor and record: VS, UO, I/O, neurovital signs
    e. Administer medications
    f. Encourage ventilation of feelings about change in body image
    g. Maintain active and passive ROM
    h. Maintain bowel and bladder program
    i. Maintain activity as tolerated
    j. Protect from falls
    k. Maintain stress-free environment

8. Patient/family postoperative teaching goals; the patient will:
    a. Keep follow-up appointments
    b. Maintain regular exercise program
    c. State the action, side effects, and scheduling of medications
    d. Identify and reduce stress
    e. Recognize the signs and symptoms of exacerbation of illness
    f. Avoid exposure to people with infections
    g. Alternate rest periods with activity
    h. Monitor self for infection
    i. Follow dietary recommendations and restrictions
    j. Promote a safe environment
    k. Maintain a quiet environment
    l. Seek help from community agencies and resources
    m. Minimize environmental stress
    n. Use assistive devices in activities of daily living (ADL)
    o. Reinforce independence
    p. Avoid extremes of hot or cold

9. Possible medical complications
    a. Urinary tract infection
    b. Respiratory tract infection
    c. Contractures
    d. Depression
    e. Paraplegia
    f. Quadriplegia

10. Possible surgical interventions: contralateral thalamotomy

K. Myasthenia gravis

1. Definition: neuromuscular disorder that results in muscle weakness of voluntary muscles
2. Possible etiology
   a. Insufficient acetylcholine
   b. Autoimmune disease
   c. Excessive cholinesterase
3. Pathophysiology
   a. Disturbance occurs in transmission of nerve impulses at the myoneural junction
   b. Transmission defect results from deficiency in release of acetylcholine or deficient number of acetylcholine receptor sites
   c. Thymus gland may remain active, triggering autoimmune reaction
4. Possible clinical manifestations
   a. Muscle weakness that increases with activity and decreases with rest
   b. Dysphagia
   c. Diplopia
   d. Dysarthria
   e. Ptosis
   f. Strabismus
   g. Impaired speech
   h. Respiratory distress
   i. Masklike expression
   j. Drooling
5. Possible diagnostic test findings
   a. Neostigmine (Prostigmin) or edrophonium (Tensilon) test: relief of symptoms after administration of medication
   b. Electromyography: decreased amplitude of evoked potentials
   c. Thymus scan: hyperplasia or thymoma
6. Medical management
   a. Diet therapy: soft
   b. Activity: as tolerated
   c. Monitoring: VS, UO, I/O, neurovital signs
   d. Glucocorticoids: prednisone (Deltasone), dexamethasone (Decadron), corticotropin (ACTH)
   e. Antacids: magnesium and aluminum hydroxide (Maalox), aluminum hydroxide gel (Alternagel)
   f. Anticholinesterases: neostigmine (Prostigmin), pyridostigmine bromide (Mestinon), ambenonium chloride (Mytelase)
   g. Plasmapheresis
7. Medical nursing interventions/responsibilities
   a. Maintain diet
   b. Assess neurologic and respiratory status
   c. Assess swallow and gag reflexes
   d. Monitor and record VS, UO, I/O, neurovital signs
   e. Administer medications

      f. Encourage ventilation of feelings about change in body image and communication

      g. Assess patient's activity tolerance

      h. Provide rest periods

      i. Provide oral hygiene

      j. Protect from falls

      k. Monitor patient for choking while eating

  8. Patient/family postoperative teaching goals; the patient will:

      a. Keep follow-up appointments

      b. Maintain regular exercise program

      c. State the action, side effects, and scheduling of medications

      d. Identify and reduce stress

      e. Recognize the signs and symptoms of respiratory distress and myasthenic crisis

      f. Adhere to activity limitations

      g. Avoid exposure to people with infections

      h. Alternate rest periods with activity

      i. Monitor self for infection

      j. Promote a safe environment

      k. Maintain a quiet environment

      l. Seek help from community agencies and resources

      m. Minimize environmental stress

  9. Possible medical complications

      a. Myasthenic crisis: increased symptoms of muscular weakness from undermedication or stress; symptoms improve with edrophonium (Tensilon)

      b. Cholinergic crisis: increased symptoms of muscular weakness and side effects of anticholinesterase medications from overmedication with cholinergic drugs; symptoms worsen with Edrophonium (Tensilon)

 10. Possible surgical interventions: thymectomy

L. Guillain-Barré syndrome (polyradiculitis, acute infectious polyneuritis)

  1. Definition: peripheral polyneuritis characterized by ascending paralysis

  2. Possible etiology

      a. Unknown cause

      b. Virus

      c. Infection

      d. Autoimmune disease

  3. Pathophysiology

      a. Preceding infection synthesizes lymphocytes, which attack myelin sheath, causing demyelinization

      b. Demyelinization is followed by inflammation around nerve roots, veins, and capillaries

      c. Inflammatory process compresses nerve roots

4. Possible clinical manifestations
   a. Generalized weakness
   b. Paralysis that starts in legs
   c. Ascending paralysis
   d. Respiratory paralysis
   e. Tachycardia
   f. Hypertension
   g. Increased temperature
   h. Ptosis
   i. Facial weakness
   j. Dysphagia
   k. Dysarthria
5. Possible diagnostic test findings
   a. CSF analysis: increased protein
   b. EMG: slowed nerve conduction
6. Medical management
   a. Diet therapy: high-calorie, high-protein
   b. Position: semi-Fowler
   c. Activity: bed rest, active and passive ROM, isometric exercises
   d. Monitoring: VS, UO, I/O, neurovital signs
   e. Plasmapheresis
   f. Nutritional support: gastrostomy feedings, NG feedings
   g. Intubation and mechanical ventilation
   h. Physical therapy
   i. Treatments: Foley catheter, chest physiotherapy (CPT), postural drainage, suction
   j. Antibiotics: amoxicillin (Amoxil), ampicillin (Omnipen), gentamicin (Garamycin)
   k. Glucocorticoids: prednisone (Deltasone), dexamethasone (Decadron), corticotropin (ACTH)
   l. Antacids: magnesium and aluminum hydroxide (Maalox), aluminum hydroxide gel (Alternagel)
   m. Turn every 2 hours
7. Medical nursing interventions/responsibilities
   a. Maintain diet
   b. Administer oxygen
   c. Provide pulmonary toilet: suction, TCDB
   d. Assess respiratory and neurologic status
   e. Maintain position, patency of NG and endotracheal tube
   f. Maintain semi-Fowler position
   g. Monitor and record VS, UO, I/O, neurovital signs
   h. Administer medications
   i. Encourage ventilation of feelings about change in body image and communication, powerlessness
   j. Assess muscle strength

    k. Assess gag and swallow reflexes
    l. Provide eye and mouth care
    m. Establish means of communication
    n. Protect from falls
    o. Prevent skin breakdown
    p. Provide ROM
    q. Assess for Homans' sign
    r. Provide bowel and bladder program
    s. Apply antiembolitic stockings
8. Patient/family teaching goals; the patient will:
    a. Keep follow-up appointments
    b. Stop smoking
    c. State the action, side effects, and scheduling of medications
    d. Identify and reduce stress
    e. Recognize the signs and symptoms of respiratory distress
    f. Avoid exposure to people with infections
    g. Alternate rest periods with activity
    h. Monitor self for infection
    i. Follow dietary recommendations and restrictions
    j. Promote a safe environment
    k. Maintain a quiet environment
    l. Seek help from community agencies and resources
    m. Minimize environmental stress
    n. Maintain regular exercise program for hands, arms, and legs
9. Possible medical complications
    a. Respiratory failure
    b. Contractures
    c. Aspiration
    d. Pneumonia
10. Possible surgical interventions: none

M. Seizure disorders
1. Definition
    a. Abnormal discharge of electrical impulses from nerve cells that results in involuntary muscle contractions
    b. International classification of seizures includes three types: partial (Jacksonian, psychomotor); generalized (petit mal, clonic, tonic); unilateral
2. Possible etiology
    a. Idiopathic
    b. Head injury
    c. Hypoglycemia
    d. Brain tumor
    e. Infection
    f. Anoxia

3. Pathophysiology
   a. Many neurons fire in synchronous pattern, resulting in transient physiologic disturbance
   b. Physiologic disturbances include change in level of consciousness, abnormal movements, and abnormal sensations
4. Possible clinical manifestations
   a. Aura
   b. Loss of consciousness
   c. Dyspnea
   d. Fixed and dilated pupils
   e. Incontinence
5. Possible diagnostic test findings
   a. EEG: abnormal wave patterns, focus of seizure activity
   b. CT scan: presence of space-occupying lesion
6. Medical management
   a. Diet therapy: ketogenic
   b. I.V. therapy: heparin lock
   c. Activity: bed rest
   d. Monitoring: VS, UO, I/O, neurovital signs
   e. Laboratory studies: glucose, potassium, Dilantin levels
   f. Precautions: seizure
   g. Anticonvulsants: phenytoin sodium (Dilantin), ethosuximide (Zarontin), phenobarbital (Luminal), diazepam (Valium)
7. Medical nursing interventions/responsibilities
   a. Maintain diet
   b. Assess neurologic and respiratory status
   c. Monitor and record VS, UO, I/O, neurovital signs, laboratory studies
   d. Administer medications
   e. Encourage ventilation of feelings about powerlessness
   f. Maintain seizure precautions
   g. Protect the patient during seizure activity
   h. Observe and record seizure activity: initial movement, respiratory pattern, length of seizure, loss of consciousness, aura, incontinence, pupillary changes
   i. Assess postictal state
   j. Maintain airway
   k. Protect patient from falls
8. Patient/family teaching goals; the patient will:
   a. Keep follow-up appointments
   b. State the action, side effects, and scheduling of medications
   c. Identify and reduce stress
   d. Recognize the signs and symptoms of seizure activity
   e. Adhere to activity limitations
   f. Avoid use of alcohol
   g. Alternate rest periods with activity
   h. Follow dietary recommendations and restrictions

      i. Promote a safe environment
      j. Seek help from community agencies and resources
      k. Wear a medical identification bracelet
      l. Identify and time seizure activity
      m. Prevent injury during seizure activity

9. Possible medical complications
   a. Musculoskeletal injury
   b. Hypoxia
   c. Status epilepticus
10. Possible surgical interventions: excision of epileptogenic area (rare)

N. Increased ICP
1. Definition: elevated ICP beyond the normal pressure exerted by blood, brain, and CSF within the skull
2. Possible etiology
   a. Tumor
   b. Abscess
   c. Space-occupying lesion
   d. Edema
   e. Hemorrhage
   f. Hydrocephalus
   g. Head injury
3. Pathophysiology
   a. Because the skull cannot expand, an increase in brain tissue, CSF, or blood results in increased ICP
   b. Increased ICP results in decreased cerebral circulation and anoxia, which can lead to permanent brain damage
4. Possible clinical manifestations
   a. Restlessness
   b. Hypotension
   c. Bradycardia
   d. Pupillary changes: sluggish reaction, dilatation
   e. Weakness
   f. Decreased level of consciousness
   g. Widening pulse pressure
   h. Abnormal posturing: decortication, decerebration
   i. Headache
   j. Vomiting
   k. Papilledema
5. Possible diagnostic test findings
   a. ICP measurement via ventriculostomy, epidural sensor, and subarachnoid screw: increased pressure
   b. LP: contraindicated
6. Medical management
   a. Diet therapy: withhold food and fluids; restrict fluids only
   b. I.V. therapy: electrolyte replacement, heparin lock

    c. Oxygen therapy
    d. Intubation and mechanical ventilation with hyperventilation
    e. Gastrointestinal decompression: NG tube
    f. Position: semi-Fowler
    g. Activity: bedrest, passive ROM
    h. Monitoring: VS, UO, I/O, EKG, ICP, neurovital signs, arterial pressure
    i. Laboratory studies: potassium, sodium, glucose, osmolality, BUN, Cr
    j. Treatments: Foley catheter
    k. ICP monitoring: ventriculostomy, subarachnoid screw, epidural sensor
    l. Diuretics: mannitol (Osmitrol), furosemide (Lasix)
    m. Antacids: magnesium and aluminum hydroxide (Maalox)
    n. CSF drainage via ventriculostomy
    o. Anticonvulsants: phenytoin sodium (Dilantin)
    p. Glucocorticoids: dexamethasone (Decadron)
    q. Histamine antagonists: cimetidine (Tagamet), ranitidine (Zantac)
    r. Barbiturate-induced coma
    s. Precautions: seizure

7. Medical nursing interventions/responsibilities
    a. Maintain fluid restriction
    b. Administer I.V. fluids
    c. Administer oxygen
    d. Provide pulmonary toilet: suction, TCDB
    e. Assess neurologic and respiratory status
    f. Maintain position, patency, low suction of NG tube
    g. Maintain position and patency of ET and Foley catheter
    h. Maintain semi-Fowler position
    i. Monitor and record VS, UO, I/O, ICP, neurovital signs, laboratory studies
    j. Administer medications
    k. Allay anxiety
    l. Maintain neutral alignment
    m. Turn every 2 hours
    n. Prevent jugular venous constriction
    o. Allow a period of rest between each nursing activity
    p. Maintain a quiet environment
    q. Maintain bed rest
    r. Prevent Valsalva's maneuver
    s. Provide mouth and skin care
    t. Provide appropriate sensory input and stimuli with frequent reorientation
    u. Assist with ADL
    v. Maintain seizure precautions

8. Patient/family teaching goals; the patient will:
    a. Keep follow-up appointments
    b. Maintain regular exercise program
    c. State the action, side effects, and scheduling of medications

    d. Recognize the signs and symptoms of decreased level of consciousness and seizures

    e. Alternate rest periods with activity

    f. Promote a safe environment

    g. Maintain a quiet environment

    h. Seek help from community agencies and resources

    i. Minimize environmental stress

    j. Set limits for impulsive behavior

    k. Adhere to fluid restrictions

    l. Identify and reduce stress

    m. Adhere to activity limitations

9. Possible medical complications

    a. Tentorial herniation

    b. Herniation through foramen magnum

    c. Death

    d. Coma

    e. Seizure

10. Possible surgical interventions: craniotomy for surgical decompression (see page 83)

O. Head injury

1. Definition

    a. Classified by the type of fracture, hemorrhage, or trauma to the brain

    b. Fractures: depressed, comminuted, or linear

    c. Hemorrhages: epidural, subdural, intracerebral, or subarachnoid

    d. Trauma: concussion, contusion

2. Possible etiology

    a. Auto accidents

    b. Falls

    c. Assaults

    d. Blunt trauma

    e. Penetrating trauma

3. Pathophysiology: brain injury or bleeding within the brain results in edema and hypoxia

4. Possible clinical manifestations

    a. Disorientation to time, place, or person

    b. Paresthesia

    c. Positive Babinski reflex

    d. Decreased level of consciousness

    e. Otorrhea

    f. Rhinorrhea

    g. Unequal pupil size

    h. Loss of pupil reaction

5. Possible diagnostic test findings

    a. Skull X-ray: skull fracture

    b. CT scan: hemorrhage, cerebral edema, or shift of midline structures

   c. MRI: hemorrhage, cerebral edema, or shift of midline structures

   d. Cerebral angiography: intracerebral, subdural, epidural hematoma

   e. Echoencephalogram: shift of midline structures

 6. Medical management

   a. Diet therapy: restrict fluid intake

   b. I.V. therapy: electrolyte replacement; heparin lock

   c. Oxygen therapy

   d. Intubation and mechanical ventilation with hyperventilation

   e. Gastrointestinal decompression: NG tube

   f. Position: semi-Fowler

   g. Activity: bed rest, active and passive ROM

   h. Monitoring: VS, UO, I/O, EKG, hemodynamic variables, ICP, CVP, neurovital signs, arterial line

   i. Laboratory studies: potassium, sodium, osmolality, arterial blood gases (ABGs), Hgb, Hct

   j. Treatments: Foley catheter

   k. Analgesics: codeine (Paveral)

   l. Diuretics: mannitol (Osmitrol), furosemide (Lasix)

   m. Antacids: magnesium and aluminum hydroxide (Maalox), aluminum hydroxide gel (Alternagel)

   n. Anticonvulsants: phenytoin sodium (Dilantin)

   o. Glucocorticoids: dexamethasone (Decadron)

   p. Histamine antagonists: cimetidine (Tagamet), ranitidine (Zantac)

   q. Cervical collar

   r. Reflex checks: oculocephalic, oculovestibular, corneal, cough, gag

 7. Medical nursing interventions/responsibilities

   a. Maintain fluid restrictions

   b. Administer I.V. fluids

   c. Administer oxygen

   d. Provide pulmonary toilet: suction, TCDB

   e. Assess neurologic and respiratory status

   f. Maintain position, patency, low suction of NG tube

   g. Maintain position and patency of ET and Foley catheter

   h. Maintain semi-Fowler position

   i. Monitor and record VS, UO, I/O, hemodynamic variables, ICP, CVP, specific gravity, urine glucose and ketones, laboratory studies

   j. Maintain seizure precautions

   k. Administer medications

   l. Encourage ventilation of feelings about change in body image

   m. Assess for CSF leak: otorrhea, rhinorrhea

   n. Assess pain

   o. Assess for diabetes insipidus

   p. Check cough and gag reflex

   q. Provide appropriate sensory input and stimuli with frequent reorientation

   r. Provide means of communication

   s. Assess for signs of increasing ICP

      t. Provide eye, skin, and mouth care
      u. Turn every 2 hours
      v. Assist with ADL
  8. Patient/family teaching goals; the patient will:
      a. Keep follow-up appointments
      b. Maintain regular exercise program
      c. State the action, side effects, and scheduling of medications
      d. Recognize the signs and symptoms of decreased level of consciousness and seizures
      e. Alternate rest periods with activity
      f. Promote a safe environment
      g. Maintain a quiet environment
      h. Seek help from community agencies and resources
      i. Minimize environmental stress
      j. Set limits for impulsive behavior
      k. Adhere to fluid restrictions
  9. Possible medical complications
      a. Shock
      b. Meningitis
      c. Increased ICP
      d. Stress ulcer
      e. Diabetes insipidus
      f. Infection
10. Possible surgical interventions: craniotomy for evacuation of hematomas (see page 83)

P. Cerebrovascular accident (CVA)
  1. Definition: disruption of cerebral circulation that results in motor and sensory deficits
  2. Possible etiology
      a. Cerebral arteriosclerosis
      b. Syphilis
      c. Trauma
      d. Hypertension
      e. Thrombosis
      f. Embolism
      g. Hemorrhage
      h. Vasospasm
  3. Pathophysiology
      a. Disruption of cerebral blood flow causes cerebral anoxia
      b. Cerebral anoxia results in cerebral infarction
      c. Infarction results in edema
  4. Possible clinical manifestations
      a. Syncope
      b. Change in level of consciousness
      c. Paresthesia

      d. Headache

      e. Aphasia

      f. Seizures

      g. Labile emotional responses

      h. Paralysis

5. Possible diagnostic test findings

      a. LP: increased pressure, bloody CSF

      b. CT scan: intracranial bleeding, infarct, or shift of midline structures

      c. EEG: focal slowing in area of lesion

      d. MRI: intracranial bleeding, infarct, or shift of midline structures

      e. Brain scan: decreased perfusion

      f. Digital subtraction angiography: occlusion or narrowing of vessels

6. Medical management

      a. Diet therapy: low-sodium

      b. I.V. therapy: heparin lock

      c. Oxygen therapy

      d. Intubation and mechanical ventilation

      e. Gastrointestinal decompression: NG tube

      f. Position: semi-Fowler

      g. Activity: bed rest, active and passive ROM, isometric exercises

      h. Monitoring: VS, UO, I/O, EKG, ICP, neurovital signs

      i. Laboratory studies: sodium, potassium, glucose, ABGs, PT, PTT

      j. Nutritional support: IVH

      k. Treatments: Foley catheter, incentive spirometry

      l. Precautions: seizure

      m. Analgesics: codeine (Paveral)

      n. Diuretics: mannitol (Osmitrol), furosemide (Lasix)

      o. Antacids: magnesium and aluminum hydroxide (Maalox), aluminum hydroxide gel (Alternagel)

      p. Anticonvulsants: phenytoin sodium (Dilantin)

      q. Glucocorticoids: dexamethasone (Decadron)

      r. Histamine antagonists: cimetidine (Tagamet), ranitidine (Zantac)

      s. Antihypertensives: diazoxide (Hyperstat)

      t. Anticoagulants: warfarin sodium (Coumadin)

      u. Physical therapy

7. Medical nursing interventions/responsibilities

      a. Maintain diet

      b. Administer I.V. fluids

      c. Administer oxygen

      d. Provide pulmonary toilet: suction, TCDB

      e. Assess neurovascular, cardiac, and respiratory status

      f. Maintain position, patency, low suction of NG tube

      g. Maintain semi-Fowler position

      h. Monitor and record VS, UO, I/O, ICP, neurovital signs, laboratory studies

      i. Administer IVH

       j. Administer medications
       k. Encourage ventilation of feelings about change in body image and difficulty communicating
       l. Maintain a quiet environment
      m. Assess for receptive/expressive aphasia
       n. Assess for hemianopsia
       o. Protect from falls and injury
       p. Apply antiembolitic stockings
       q. Maintain seizure precautions
       r. Provide passive ROM
       s. Turn and position every 2 hours
       t. Provide means of communication
       u. Provide skin and mouth care

8. Patient/family teaching goals; the patient will:
       a. Keep follow-up appointments
       b. Maintain regular exercise program
       c. Stop smoking
       d. Maintain ideal weight
       e. State the action, side effects, and scheduling of medications
       f. Identify and reduce stress
       g. Recognize the signs and symptoms of seizures
       h. Adhere to activity limitations
       i. Alternate rest periods with activity
       j. Follow dietary recommendations and restrictions
       k. Promote a safe environment
       l. Maintain a quiet environment
      m. Seek help from community agencies and resources
       n. Minimize environmental stress
       o. Reinforce established methods of communication with the aphasic patient
       p. Monitor blood pressure
       q. Use assistive devices in ADL

9. Possible medical complications
       a. Cerebral edema
       b. Vasospasm
       c. Pneumonia
       d. Increased ICP
       e. Complications of immobility: thrombophlebitis, pulmonary embolism, osteoporosis, urinary stasis

10. Possible surgical interventions
       a. Carotid endarterectomy (see page 85)
       b. Craniotomy for evacuation of clot (see page 83)

Q. Cerebral aneurysm
1. Definition
       a. Dilatation or localized weakness of the middle layer of an artery
       b. Classified by types: saccular (berry), fusiform, and mycotic

2. Possible etiology
   a. Atherosclerosis
   b. Trauma
   c. Congenital weakness
   d. Syphilis
3. Pathophysiology
   a. Enlargement of aneurysm compresses nerves
   b. Enlargement of the aneurysm finally results in dissolution of the wall and rupture of the aneurysm
   c. Rupture of the aneurysm results in subarachnoid hemorrhage
   d. Release of serotonin, prostaglandins, and catecholamines from blood precipitates vasospasm
4. Possible clinical manifestations
   a. Diplopia
   b. Ptosis
   c. Headache
   d. Hemiparesis
   e. Nuchal rigidity
   f. Decreased level of consciousness
   g. Seizure activity
   h. Blurred vision
5. Possible diagnostic test findings
   a. CT scan: shift of intracranial midline structures, blood in subarachnoid space
   b. MRI: shift of intracranial midline structures, blood in subarachnoid space
   c. Cerebral angiogram: identification of vasospasm and vasculature associated with aneurysm
   d. LP (contraindicated with increased ICP): increased pressure, protein, WBC; bloody and xanthochromic CSF
6. Medical management
   a. I.V. therapy: heparin lock
   b. Oxygen therapy
   c. Position: semi-Fowler
   d. Activity: bed rest, passive ROM
   e. Monitoring: VS, UO, I/O, ICP, neurovital signs, arterial line
   f. Precautions: aneurysm and seizure
   g. Antacids: magnesium and aluminum hydroxide (Maalox), aluminum hydroxide gel (Alternagel)
   h. Anticonvulsants: phenytoin sodium (Dilantin)
   i. Glucocorticoids: dexamethasone (Decadron)
   j. Histamine antagonists: cimetidine (Tagamet), ranitidine (Zantac)
   k. Stool softeners: docusate sodium (Colace)
   l. Antifibrolytics: aminocaproic acid (Amicar)
   m. Antihypertensives: methylodopa (Aldomet), hydralazine (Apresoline)
   n. Ergot alkaloid: methysergide (Sansert)

7. Medical nursing interventions/responsibilities
   a. Maintain fluid restriction
   b. Administer oxygen
   c. Assess neurologic status
   d. Maintain semi-Fowler position
   e. Monitor and record VS, UO, I/O, ICP
   f. Administer medication
   g. Encourage ventilation of feelings about fear of dying
   h. Allay anxiety
   i. Maintain a quiet, darkened environment
   j. Assess pain
   k. Allow a rest period between nursing activities
   l. Maintain bed rest
   m. Prevent Valsalva's maneuver
   n. Assess for signs of increased ICP
   o. Maintain seizure and aneurysm precautions
   p. Provide passive ROM
   q. Limit visitors
   r. Provide skin care
   s. Assist with ADL
   t. Prevent constipation
   u. Assess for meningeal irritation
8. Patient/family teaching goals; the patient will:
   a. Keep follow-up appointments
   b. State the action, side effects, and scheduling of medications
   c. Identify and reduce stress
   d. Recognize the signs and symptoms of decreasing level of consciousness and seizures
   e. Adhere to activity limitations
   f. Promote a safe environment
   g. Maintain a quiet environment
   h. Minimize environmental stress
   i. Alter ADL to compensate for neurologic deficits
   j. Prevent constipation
9. Possible medical complications
   a. Vasospasm
   b. Rebleed of the aneurysm
   c. Increased ICP
   d. Rupture of the aneurysm
   e. Hydrocephalus
   f. Brain herniation
10. Possible surgical interventions
   a. Craniotomy for clipping or wrapping of aneurysm (see page 83)
   b. Craniotomy for evacuation of hematoma (see page 83)

R. Brain tumor
1. Definition: malignant or benign tumor of the brain that may be primary or metastatic
2. Possible etiology
   a. Genetic
   b. Environmental
3. Pathophysiology
   a. Unregulated cell growth and uncontrolled cell division result in the development of a neoplasm
   b. Tumors are classified according to tissue of origin: gliomas, meningiomas, metastatic
   c. Tumors can be infiltrative and destroy surrounding tissue or be encapsulated and displace brain tissue
   d. Presence of lesion and compression of blood vessels produces ischemia, edema, and increased ICP
4. Possible clinical manifestations
   a. Headache
   b. Vomiting
   c. Papilledema
   d. Frontal tumor: personality changes, aphasia, memory loss, headache
   e. Temporal tumor: seizures, aphasia, headache
   f. Parietal tumor: motor seizures, sensory impairment
   g. Occipital tumor: visual impairment, homonymous hemianopsia, visual hallucinations
   h. Cerebellar tumor: impairment of equilibrium and coordination
5. Possible diagnostic test findings
   a. EEG: seizure activity
   b. CT scan: location and size of tumor
   c. Skull X-ray: location and size of tumor
   d. Angiography: location and size of tumor
   e. LP (contraindicated with increased ICP): increased protein
6. Medical management
   a. Diet therapy: high-protein, high-calorie
   b. I.V. therapy: heparin lock
   c. Oxygen therapy
   d. Position: semi-Fowler
   e. Activity: bed rest
   f. Monitoring: VS, UO, I/O, ICP, neurovital signs
   g. Laboratory studies: sodium, potassium glucose
   h. Nutritional support: IVH
   i. Radiation therapy
   j. Antineoplastics: vincristine sulfate (Oncovin), lomustine (CCNU), carmustine (BiCNU)
   k. Diuretics: mannitol (Osmitrol), furosemide (Lasix)
   l. Antacids: magnesium and aluminum hydroxide (Maalox), aluminum hydroxide gel (Alternagel)

    m. Anticovulsants: phenytoin sodium (Dilantin)

    n. Glucocorticoids: dexamethasone (Decadron)

    o. Histamine antagonists: cimetidine (Tagamet), ranitidine (Zantac)

    p. Precautions: seizure

    q. Chemotherapy

7. Medical nursing interventions/responsibilities
   a. Maintain diet
   b. Encourage fluids
   c. Administer I.V. fluids
   d. Administer oxygen
   e. Assess neurologic and respiratory status
   f. Maintain semi-Fowler position
   g. Monitor and record VS, UO, I/O, ICP, neurovital signs, laboratory studies
   h. Administer IVH
   i. Administer medications
   j. Encourage ventilation of feelings about change in body image and fear of dying
   k. Assess pain
   l. Assess for increased ICP
   m. Provide oral hygiene
   n. Provide postchemotherapeutic and/or postradiation nursing care: provide skin, mouth, and perineal care; encourage dietary intake; administer antiemetics and antidiarrheals; monitor for bleeding, infection, and electrolyte imbalance; provide rest periods
   o. Maintain seizure precautions

8. Patient/family teaching goals; the patient will:
   a. Keep follow-up appointments
   b. Maintain regular exercise program
   c. Maintain ideal weight
   d. State the action, side effects, and scheduling of medications
   e. Identify and reduce stress
   f. Recognize the signs and symptoms of change in level of consciousness
   g. Adhere to activity limitations
   h. Avoid exposure to people with infections
   i. Alternate rest periods with activity
   j. Monitor self for infection
   k. Follow dietary recommendations and restrictions
   l. Promote a safe environment
   m. Maintain a quiet environment

9. Possible medical complications
   a. Increased ICP
   b. Brain herniation
   c. Seizures

10. Possible surgical interventions: craniotomy for surgical excision of tumor (see page 83)

S. Spinal cord injury

1. Definition
   a. Traumatic injury to the spinal cord that results in sensory and motor deficits
   b. Types: paraplegia, quadriplegia
2. Possible etiology
   a. Car accidents
   b. Falls
   c. Gunshot wounds
   d. Stab wounds
   e. Diving into shallow water
   f. Infections
   g. Tumors
   h. Congenital anomalies
3. Pathophysiology
   a. Injury may result in complete transection of the spinal cord
   b. Associated edema and hemorrhage from the injury cause ischemia
   c. Necrosis and scar tissue form in the area of the traumatized cord
   d. Paraplegia is paralysis of the legs
   e. Quadriplegia is paralysis of all four extremities
4. Possible clinical manifestations
   a. Paralysis below the level of the injury
   b. Paresthesia below the level of the injury
   c. Neck pain
   d. Loss of bowel and bladder control
   e. Respiratory distress
   f. Numbness and tingling
   g. Flaccid muscle
   h. Absence of reflexes below level of the injury
5. Possible diagnostic test findings
   a. Spinal X-rays: vertebral fracture
   b. CT scan: spinal cord edema, vertebral fracture, spinal cord compression
   c. MRI: spinal cord edema, vertebral fracture, spinal cord compression
6. Medical management
   a. Diet therapy: low-calcium, high-protein
   b. I.V. therapy: heparin lock
   c. Oxygen therapy
   d. Intubation and mechanical ventilation
   e. Gastrointestinal decompression: NG tube
   f. Position: flat
   g. Activity: bed rest, passive ROM
   h. Monitoring: VS, UO, I/O, EKG, ICP, neurovital signs
   i. Laboratory studies: sodium, potassium, glucose, WBC
   j. Treatments: Foley catheter
   k. Antacids: magnesium and aluminum hydroxide (Maalox), aluminum hydroxide gel (Alternagel)

l. Anticonvulsants: phenytoin sodium (Dilantin)
m. Glucocorticoids: dexamethasone (Decadron)
n. Histamine antagonists: cimetidine (Tagamet), ranitidine (Zantac)
o. Cervical collar
p. Maintenance of vertebral aligment: Stryker turning frame, Crutchfield tongs, Halo brace
q. Laxatives: bisacodyl (Dulcolax)
r. Antianxiety agents: diazepam (Valium)
s. Antihypertensives: diazoxide (Hyperstat), hydralazine (Apresoline)
t. Muscle relaxants: dantrolene sodium (Dantrium)
7. Medical nursing interventions/responsibilities
   a. Maintain diet
   b. Force fluids
   c. Administer I.V. fluids
   d. Administer oxygen
   e. Provide pulmonary toilet: suction, TCDB
   f. Assess neurologic and respiratory status
   g. Maintain flat position
   h. Monitor and record VS, UO, I/O, laboratory studies
   i. Administer medications
   j. Encourage ventilation of feelings about change in body image, change in sexual expression and function, altered mobility
   k. Turn every 2 hours using logrolling technique
   l. Maintain body alignment
   m. Initiate bowel and bladder retraining
   n. Provide sexual counseling
   o. Provide passive ROM
   p. Assess for autonomic dysreflexia
   q. Assess for spinal shock
   r. Provide skin care
   s. Provide heel and elbow protectors and sheepskin
   t. Apply antiembolitic stockings
8. Patient/family teaching goals; the patient will:
   a. Keep follow-up appointments
   b. Maintain regular exercise program for muscle building
   c. Maintain ideal weight
   d. State the action, side effects, and scheduling of medications
   e. Identify and reduce stress
   f. Recognize the signs and symptoms of autonomic dysreflexia, urinary tract infection, upper respiratory infection
   g. Monitor self for infection
   h. Follow dietary recommendations and restrictions
   i. Promote a safe environment
   j. Seek help from community agencies and resources
   k. Maintain bowel and bladder program
   l. Maintain acidic urine with cranberry juice

     m. Maintain adequate fluid intake: 3,000 ml/day
     n. Use assistive devices for ADL
     o. Maintain skin integrity
     p. Maintain mobility using a wheelchair
     q. Reinforce independence
9. Possible medical complications
     a. Spinal shock
     b. Autonomic dysreflexia
     c. Respiratory distress
10. Possible surgical interventions
     a. Laminectomy (see page 54)
     b. Spinal cord fusion (see page 55)

Points to Remember

Environmental stress and sensory stimulation should be limited for the patient with a nervous system disorder.

In managing a patient with a nervous system disorder, the focus of the health-care team is to optimize and maintain the highest level of function.

Nursing assessment should focus on changes in the level of consciousness and signs of increasing intracranial pressure for patients with nervous system disorders that include brain involvement.

Alternate methods of communication need to be established to prepare patients for progressive debilitation in nervous system disorders.

Powerlessness, change in body image, and lowered self-esteem are central themes in a patient's response to nervous system disorders.

Glossary

Ataxia — lack of muscular coordination.

Decerebrate posturing — abnormal extension and internal rotation of arms and legs.

Neurovital signs — evaluation of neurologic status that may include assessment of pupils, motor and verbal response, level of consciousness, vital signs, pulse pressure, mean arterial pressure, and intracranial pressure.

Papilledema — swelling of the optic nerve head.

Ptosis — drooping of the eyelid.

Gastrointestinal System

Learning Objectives
After studying this section, the reader should be able to:

• Describe the psychosocial impact of gastrointestinal system disorders.

• Differentiate between modifiable and nonmodifiable risk factors in the development of a gastrointestinal system disorder.

• List three potential and three actual nursing diagnoses for the patient with a gastrointestinal system disorder.

• Identify the medical and surgical nursing interventions/responsibilities for the patient with a gastrointestinal system disorder.

• Write three teaching goals for the patient with a gastrointestinal system disorder.

IV. Gastrointestinal System

A. Anatomy and physiology

1. Mouth
   a. Mechanical and chemical digestion originate here
   b. Tongue and teeth are accessory organs of digestion
   c. Salivary glands secrete saliva, which combines with food during mastication
2. Esophagus
   a. This organ provides for transfer of food from the oropharynx to the stomach
   b. The closure of the epiglottis prevents food from entering the trachea
   c. Closure of the cardiac sphincter prevents reflux of gastric contents
3. Stomach
   a. Is hollow, one-liter muscular pouch
   b. Secretes pepsin, renin, lipase, mucus, hydrochloric acid, and intrinsic factor for digestion
   c. Mixes and stores chyme
4. Small intestine
   a. It consists of duodenum, jejunum, and ileum
   b. Chyme enters the duodenum through the pyloric sphincter
   c. It is the site of digestion and absorption of nutrients
   d. Bile and pancreatic secretions enter the duodenum through the common bile duct at the ampulla of Vater
   e. It is lined with villi that contain capillaries and lymphatics
   f. Chyme is liquid or semiliquid
   g. Motor activity includes mixing and peristalsis
5. Large intestine
   a. It consists of cecum, colon, rectum, and anus
   b. Segments of the colon are the cecum, ascending colon, transverse colon, descending colon, and sigmoid colon
   c. Chyme enters cecum through the ileocecal valve
   d. Functions include absorption of fluid and electrolytes; synthesis of vitamin K by intestinal bacteria; storage of fecal material
   e. Chyme becomes more solid as water is absorbed through the intestinal wall of the colon
   f. Defecation is the movement of feces from the rectum through the anal sphincter
6. Liver
   a. Is largest organ in the body
   b. Produces bile (main function) which emulsifies fats and stimulates peristalsis
   c. Conveys bile to the duodenum, where it enters at the sphincter of Oddi through the common bile duct
   d. Metabolizes carbohydrates, fats, and proteins
   e. Synthesizes coagulation factors VII, IX, X and prothrombin

      f. Stores vitamins A, D, B_{12}, and iron
      g. Detoxifies chemicals
      h. Excretes bilirubin
      i. Receives dual blood supply from portal vein and hepatic artery
      j. Produces and stores glycogen
      k. Promotes erythropoiesis when bone marrow production is insufficient
  7. Gall bladder
      a. Hollow, pear-shaped organ that stores bile
      b. Secretes bile via the cystic duct to the common bile duct
  8. Pancreas
      a. Accessory gland of digestion
      b. Exocrine function: secretion of digestive enzymes (amylase, lipase, and trypsin)
      c. Endocrine function: secretion of insulin, glucagon, somatostatin, and hormones (gastrin, secretin, cholecystokinin, and gastric inhibitory peptide) from islets of Langerhans
      d. Main pancreatic duct joins the common bile duct and empties into the duodenum at the ampulla of Vater

B. Physical assessment findings
  1. Subjective data that often accompany gastrointestinal (GI) disorders
      a. Diet history
      b. Change in bowel habits: constipation, diarrhea, and flatus
      c. Compaints of indigestion
      d. Change in weight
      e. Nausea and vomiting
      f. Abdominal pain
      g. Difficulty swallowing
      h. Loss of appetite
  2. Objective data to evaluate in GI disorders
      a. Dysphagia
      b. Color and consistency of stool: melena, clay, frothy, steatorrhea
      c. Quality of bowel sounds
      d. Abdominal distention
      e. Rectal bleeding
      f. Jaundice
      g. Edema
      h. Hematemesis
      i. Anorexia

C. Diagnostic tests and procedures used to evaluate GI disorders
  1. Upper GI series
      a. Definition/purpose: fluoroscopic examination of the esophagus, stomach, duodenum, and other portions of the small bowel after swallowing contrast medium (barium)

    b. Nursing interventions/responsibilities: before procedure, withhold food and fluids; administer fluids, cathartics, and enemas as ordered; after procedure, inform patient that stool will be light-colored for several days; administer cathartics, fluids, and enemas as ordered

2. Lower GI series (barium enema)

    a. Definition/purpose: fluoroscopic examination of the large intestine after administration of a contrast medium (barium) via an enema

    b. Nursing interventions/responsibilities: before procedure, withhold food and fluids; encourage patient to discuss feelings of embarrassment; administer bowel preparation (laxatives/enemas) as ordered; after procedure, assess for constipation; force fluids unless contraindicated; administer enemas and laxatives as ordered

3. Endoscopy

    a. Definition/purpose: direct visualization of the esophagus and stomach using an endoscope

    b. Nursing interventions/responsibilities: before procedure, withhold food and fluids; obtain written, informed consent; obtain baseline vital signs; administer sedatives as ordered; after procedure, withhold food and fluids until gag reflex returns; assess gag and cough reflex; assess vasovagal response

4. Fecal occult blood test

    a. Definition/purpose: analysis of stool for blood using a reagent

    b. Nursing interventions/responsibilities: before procedure, advise patient to avoid red meat, iron, and high fiber for 1 to 3 days; document the adminstration of aspirin, vitamin C, and anti-inflammatory drugs

5. Fecal fat

    a. Definition/purpose: analysis of stool for fat using a stain

    b. Nursing interventions/responsibilities: before procedure, advise the patient to restrict alcohol intake and maintain a high-fat diet 72 hours before the exam; refrigerate specimen; document current medications

6. Proctosigmoidoscopy

    a. Definition/purpose: direct visualization of the sigmoid colon, rectum, and anal canal using a lighted scope

    b. Nursing interventions/responsibilities: before procedure, encourage patient to discuss feelings of embarrassment; inform patient that he will assume a knee-chest position; administer bowel preparation as ordered; obtain written, informed consent; document iron intake; after procedure, assess for bleeding; monitor vital signs (VS)

7. Barium swallow

    a. Definition/purpose: fluoroscopic examination of pharynx and esophagus after administration of a contrast medium (barium)

    b. Nursing interventions/responsibilities: before procedure, withhold food and fluids; after procedure, assess for constipation; force fluids unless contraindicated; administer laxatives as ordered

8. Cholangiography
   a. Definition/purpose: radiographic examination of the biliary duct system after injection of radiopaque dye through a catheter
   b. Nursing interventions/responsibilities: before procedure, encourage low-residue, high-simple fat diet 1 day before the exam; withhold food and fluid after midnight; assess allergies to radiopaque dye, seafood, and iodine; inform patient he may feel flushing of the face and throat irritation; after procedure, assess insertion site for bleeding; monitor VS
9. Liver scan
   a. Definition/purpose: visual imaging of distribution of blood flow in the liver after I.V. injection of a radioisotope
   b. Nursing interventions/responsibilities: assess patient's ability to lie still during the procedure
10. Gastric analysis
    a. Definition/purpose: fasting analysis of gastric secretions by aspirating stomach contents through a nasogastric (NG) tube to measure acidity
    b. Nursing interventions/responsibilities: before procedure, withhold food and fluids; instruct patient not to smoke 8 to 12 hours before the test; withhold medications that can affect gastric secretions; after procedure, obtain VS; assess for reactions to gastric acid stimulant if used
11. Ultrasonography
    a. Definition/purpose: noninvasive examination that uses echoes from sound waves to visualize body organs
    b. Nursing interventions/responsibilities: before procedure, withhold food and fluids for 8 to 12 hours; assess patient's ability to lie still during the procedure; ask patient not to smoke or chew gum; administer enemas as ordered; remove abdominal dressings
12. Blood chemistry
    a. Definition/purpose: laboratory analysis of blood sample for potassium, sodium, calcium, phosphorus, glucose, bicarbonate, blood urea nitrogen (BUN), creatinine (Cr), protein, albumin, osmolality, amylase, lipase, alkaline phosphatase, ammonia, bilirubin, lactic dehydrogenase (LDH), bromsulphalein (BSP) test, serum glutamic oxaloacetic transaminase (SGOT), serum glutamic pyruvic transaminase (SGPT), hepatitis-associated antigens, carcinoembryonic antigen (CEA), alpha-fetoprotein (AFP)
    b. Nursing interventions/responsibilities: before procedure, withhold food and fluid as ordered; after procedure, monitor site for bleeding
13. Hematologic studies
    a. Definition/purpose: laboratory analysis of blood sample for red blood cells (RBC), white blood cells (WBC), platelets, prothrombin time (PT), partial thrombopastin time (PTT), hemoglobin (Hgb), hematocrit (Hct)
    b. Nursing interventions/responsibilities: assess site for bleeding; note current drug therapy

14. Liver biopsy
    a. Definition/purpose: percutaneous removal of a small amount of liver tissue for histologic evaluation, using a needle
    b. Nursing interventions/responsibilities: before procedure, withhold food and fluids; obtain written, informed consent; assess baseline clotting studies and VS; after procedure, assess site for bleeding; monitor vital signs; monitor patient for shock and pneumothorax

D. Possible psychosocial impact of GI disorders
1. Developmental impact
    a. Changes in body image
    b. Feeling of lack of control over body function
    c. Fear of rejection
    d. Embarrassment from change in body function and structure
    e. Decreased self-esteem
2. Economic impact
    a. Disruption of employment
    b. Cost of special diet
    c. Cost of special diversion appliances
    d. Cost of medications
3. Occupational and recreational impact
    a. Change of occupation
    b. Change in leisure activity
    c. Restrictions in physical activity
4. Social impact
    a. Change in eating patterns and modes
    b. Change in elimination patterns and modes
    c. Social withdrawal and isolation
    d. Change in sexual function

E. Possible risk factors for development of GI disorders
1. Modifiable risk factors
    a. Diet: low-fiber
    b. Cigarette smoking
    c. Alcohol consumption
    d. Inactivity
    e. Occupational stress
    f. Contaminated water and food
    g. Emotional state: anger, fear, or anxiety
2. Nonmodifiable risk factors
    a. Family history of GI disorders
    b. History of previous GI dysfunction
    c. Culturally based reluctance to discuss personal hygiene and health habits

F. Possible nursing diagnoses for the patient with a GI disorder
1. Actual nursing diagnoses
   a. Alteration in bowel elimination: constipation
   b. Alteration in bowel elimination: diarrhea
   c. Alteration in comfort: pain
   d. Alteration in nutrition: less than body requirements
   e. Fluid volume deficit: actual
2. Potential nursing diagnoses
   a. Disturbance in self-concept: body image
   b. Disturbance in self-concept: self-esteem
   c. Impairment of skin integrity: potential
   d. Self-care deficit
   e. Knowledge deficit
   f. Anxiety
   g. Sexual dysfunction

G. Surgical intervention: gall bladder and pancreatic surgeries
1. Definition
   a. Cholecystotomy: surgical incision into the gallbladder to drain bile
   b. Choledochotomy: surgical incision into the common bile duct
   c. Cholecystostomy: surgical incision into the gallbladder to remove gallstones
   d. Choledochostomy: surgical opening of the common bile duct to remove stones and insert a T tube
   e. Pancreatectomy: surgical removal of part or all of the pancreas
2. Preoperative surgical nursing interventions/responsibilities
   a. Complete patient and family preoperative teaching: assess understanding of surgical procedure; explain operating room (OR), recovery room (RR), preoperative and postoperative routine; demonstrate postoperative turning, coughing, and deep breathing (TCDB), splinting, leg exercises, and range of motion (ROM) exercises; explain postoperative need for drainage tubes, surgical dressings, oxygen therapy, I.V. therapy, and pain control
   b. Complete preoperative check list
   c. Administer preoperative medications
   d. Allay patient and family anxiety about surgery
   e. Document patient history and physical assessment data base
3. Postoperative surgical nursing interventions/responsibilities
   a. Assess respiratory status and fluid balance
   b. Assess pain and administer postoperative analgesic
   c. Progress diet as tolerated
   d. Administer I.V. fluids and transfusion therapy
   e. Allay anxiety
   f. Assess surgical dressing and change as directed
   g. Reinforce TCDB and splinting of incision
   h. Maintain semi-Fowler position

      i. Assess for return of peristalsis
      j. Provide pulmonary toilet: incentive spirometry
      k. Maintain activity as tolerated
      l. Monitor VS, urinary output (UO), intake and output (I/O), laboratory studies
      m. Monitor and maintain position and patency of drainage tubes: NG, wound drainage, T tube
      n. Administer antibiotics
      o. Pancreatic surgery: monitor urine glucose and ketones

  4. Possible surgical complications
      a. Pneumonia
      b. Atelectasis
      c. Peritonitis
      d. Hemorrhage

  5. Postoperative patient/family teaching goals; the patient will:
      a. Keep follow-up appointments
      b. Maintain regular exercise program
      c. Stop smoking
      d. Maintain ideal weight
      e. State the action, side effects, and scheduling of medications
      f. Recognize the signs and symptoms of infection
      g. Avoid lifting for 6 weeks
      h. Complete daily incision care
      i. Maintain care of the T tube
      j. Adhere to low-fat diet for 6 weeks
      k. Gall bladder surgeries: monitor color, amount, and consistency of stool
      l. Pancreatic surgery: monitor urine glucose and ketones; recognize signs of hyperglycemia

H. Surgical intervention: portal-systemic shunts

  1. Definition
      a. Portocaval shunt: surgical anastomosis of the portal vein to the inferior vena cava to divert blood from the portal system to decrease pressure
      b. Splenorenal shunt: surgical anastomosis of the splenic vein to the left renal vein to divert blood from the portal system to decrease pressure
      c. Mesocaval shunt: surgical anastomosis of the inferior vena cava to the side of the superior mesenteric vein to divert blood from the portal system to decrease pressure

  2. Preoperative surgical nursing interventions/responsibilities
      a. Complete patient and family preoperative teaching: assess understanding of surgical procedure; explain OR, RR, preoperative and postoperative routine; demonstrate postoperative TCDB, splinting, leg exercises, and ROM; explain postoperative need for drainage tubes, surgical dressings, oxygen therapy, I.V. therapy, and pain control
      b. Complete preoperative check list
      c. Administer preoperative medications

      d. Allay patient and family anxiety about surgery
      e. Document patient history and physical assessment data base
      f. Administer antibiotics
      g. Administer vitamin K
      h. Administer I.V. and transfusion therapy
      i. Administer lactulose
      j. Maintain patency of NG tube
      k. Monitor central venous pressure (CVP)

3. Postoperative surgical nursing interventions/responsibilities
      a. Assess cardiac, respiratory, and neurologic status and fluid balance
      b. Assess pain and administer postoperative analgesic
      c. Administer I.V. fluids, I.V. hyperalimentation (IVH) and transfusion therapy
      d. Allay anxiety
      e. Assess surgical dressing
      f. Reinforce TCDB and splinting of incision
      g. Maintain semi-Fowler position
      h. Assess for return of peristalsis
      i. Provide pulmonary toilet: suction
      j. Maintain activity: bed rest, active and passive ROM, isometric exercises
      k. Administer oxygen and maintain endotracheal tube to ventilator
      l. Monitor VS, UO, I/O, CVP, laboratory studies, EKG, neurovital signs
      m. Monitor and maintain position and patency of drainage tubes: NG, Foley, wound drainage
      n. Allay anxiety
      o. Measure abdominal girth
      p. Monitor stool and NG drainage for occult blood
      q. Monitor for hemorrhage
      r. Assess peripheral edema
      s. Provide skin, nares, and mouth care
      t. Reorient frequently
      u. Administer antibiotics
      v. Administer vitamin K
      w. Elevate extremities

4. Possible surgical complications
      a. Acute hepatic failure
      b. Chronic portal systemic encephalopathy
      c. Coagulopathy
      d. Shunt malfunction

5. Patient/family postoperative teaching goals; the patient will:
      a. Keep follow-up appointments
      b. Maintain regular exercise program
      c. Stop smoking
      d. Maintain ideal weight
      e. State the action, side effects, and scheduling of medications
      f. Recognize the signs and symptoms of infection

     g. Adhere to activity limitations

     h. Complete daily incision care

     i. Avoid the use of alcohol

     j. Adhere to lifelong protein-restricted diet

     k. Avoid use of over-the-counter medications

I. Surgical intervention: gastric surgery

  1. Definition

     a. Vagotomy: surgical ligation of the vagus nerve to decrease the secretion of gastric acid

     b. Antrectomy: surgical removal of the antrum of the stomach

     c. Pyloroplasty: surgical dilatation of the pyloric sphincter to increase the rate of gastric emptying

     d. Gastroduodenostomy (Bilroth I): surgical removal of the lower portion of the stomach with anastomosis of the remaining portion of the stomach to the duodenum

     e. Gastrojejunostomy (Bilroth II): surgical removal of the antrum and distal portion of the stomach and duodenum with anastomosis of the stomach to the jejunum

     f. Subtotal gastrectomy: surgical removal of 60% to 80% of the stomach

     g. Esophagojejunostomy (total gastrectomy): surgical removal of the entire stomach with a loop of the jejunum anastomosed to the esophagus

  2. Preoperative surgical nursing interventions/responsibilities

     a. Complete patient and family preoperative teaching: assess understanding of surgical procedure; explain OR, RR, preoperative and postoperative routine; demonstrate postoperative TCDB, splinting, leg exercises, and ROM; explain postoperative need for drainage tubes, surgical dressings, oxygen therapy, I.V. therapy, and pain control

     b. Complete preoperative check list

     c. Administer preoperative medications

     d. Allay patient and family anxiety about surgery

     e. Document patient history and physical assessment data base

     f. Administer bowel preparation

  3. Postoperative surgical nursing interventions/responsibilities

     a. Assess respiratory status and fluid balance

     b. Assess pain and administer postoperative analgesic

     c. Administer I.V. fluids, NG tube feedings, and transfusion therapy

     d. Allay anxiety

     e. Assess surgical dressing and change as directed

     f. Reinforce TCDB and splinting of incision

     g. Maintain semi-Fowler position

     h. Apply antiembolitic stockings

     i. Assess for return of peristalsis

     j. Provide pulmonary toilet: incentive spirometry

     k. Maintain activity: as tolerated

     l. Administer oxygen

m. Monitor VS, UO, I/O, laboratory studies
n. Monitor and maintain position and patency of drainage tubes: NG, Foley, wound drainage
o. Monitor NG drainage for overt bleeding; irrigate gently; do not reposition NG tube
p. Weigh daily
q. Monitor gastric pH
4. Possible surgical complications
a. Partial gastrectomy: dumping syndrome
b. Hemorrhage
c. Dehydration
d. Infection
e. Dehiscence
5. Patient/family postoperative teaching goals; the patient will:
a. Keep follow-up appointments
b. Maintain regular exercise program
c. Stop smoking
d. Maintain ideal weight
e. State the action, side effects, and scheduling of medications
f. Recognize the signs and symptoms of infection and dehydration
g. Complete daily incision care
h. Identify and reduce stress
i. Maintain ideal body weight
j. Increase food intake gradually
k. Adjust eating to six small meals each day
l. Limit fluids with meals

J. Surgical intervention: hemorrhoidectomy

1. Definition: surgical removal of hemorrhoids by clamp, excision, or cautery
2. Preoperative surgical nursing interventions/responsibilities
a. Complete patient and family preoperative teaching: assess understanding of surgical procedure; explain OR, RR, preoperative and postoperative routine; demonstrate postoperative TCDB, splinting, leg exercises, and ROM; explain postoperative need for drainage tubes, surgical dressings, oxygen therapy, I.V. therapy, and pain control
b. Complete preoperative check list
c. Administer preoperative medications
d. Allay patient and family anxiety about surgery
e. Document patient history and physical assessment data base
f. Administer bowel preparation of cleansing enemas and laxatives
3. Postoperative surgical nursing interventions/responsibilities
a. Assess pain and administer postoperative analgesic
b. Progress diet as tolerated
c. Administer I.V. fluids
d. Allay anxiety
e. Assess surgical dressing and remove anal packing as ordered

    f. Reinforce TCDB
    g. Maintain side-lying or prone position
    h. Assess for return of peristalsis
    i. Provide pulmonary toilet: incentive spirometry
    j. Maintain activity: as tolerated
    k. Monitor VS, UO, I/O, laboratory studies
    l. Encourage ventilation of feelings about feelings of embarrassment and fear of defecation
    m. Administer analgesics before first bowel movement
    n. Provide sitz baths
    o. Provide flotation pad when sitting
    p. Administer stool softeners
  4. Possible surgical complications
    a. Rectal hemorrhage
    b. Urinary retention
  5. Patient/family postoperative teaching goals; the patient will:
    a. Keep follow-up appointments
    b. Maintain regular exercise program
    c. Maintain ideal weight
    d. State the action, side effects, and scheduling of medications
    e. Recognize the signs and symptoms of bleeding and infection
    f. Adhere to activity limitations: avoid prolonged standing, sitting, heavy lifting
    g. Avoid constipation
    h. Defecate when urge is felt
    i. Provide daily perineal care
    j. Anticipate small amount of bleeding postoperatively with bowel movements
    k. Increase fluid intake
    l. Follow dietary recommendations and restrictions
    m. Avoid Valsalva's maneuver

K. Surgical intervention: bowel surgery

  1. Definition
    a. Abdominoperineal resection: removal of distal sigmoid colon, rectum, and anus with the creation of a permanent colostomy
    b. Colectomy: surgical excision of the right colon (right hemicolectomy) or left colon (left hemicolectomy)
    c. Ileostomy: surgical opening of the ileum onto the abdominal surface to form a stoma
    d. Continent ileostomy (Koch's pouch): surgical creation of an intra-abdominal reservoir for stool
    e. Bowel resection: surgical excision of a portion of the bowel
    f. Permanent colostomy: surgical opening of the colon onto the abdominal surface to form a single stoma after the distal portion of the bowel is removed

    g. Double barrel colostomy: surgical opening of the colon onto the abdominal surface to form two stomas to prevent passage of stool into the distal bowel

2. Preoperative surgical nursing interventions/responsibilities
   a. Complete patient and family preoperative teaching: assess understanding of surgical procedure; explain OR, RR, preoperative and postoperative routine; demonstrate postoperative TCDB, splinting, leg exercises, and ROM; explain postoperative need for drainage tubes, gastrostomy feeding tube, surgical dressings, oxygen therapy, I.V. therapy, and pain control
   b. Complete preoperative check list
   c. Administer preoperative medications
   d. Allay patient and family anxiety about surgery
   e. Document patient history and physical assessment data base
   f. Administer bowel preparation: antibiotics and cleansing enemas
   g. Administer antibiotics
   h. Arrange preoperative visit with enterostomal therapist
   i. Encourage ventilation of feelings about change in body image

3. Postoperative surgical nursing interventions/responsibilities
   a. Assess cardiac status and fluid balance
   b. Assess pain and administer postoperative analgesic
   c. Progress diet as tolerated
   d. Administer I.V. fluids, IVH, and transfusion therapy
   e. Allay anxiety
   f. Assess surgical dressing and change as directed
   g. Reinforce TCDB and splinting of incision
   h. Maintain semi-Fowler position
   i. Assess for return of peristalsis
   j. Provide pulmonary toilet: incentive spirometry
   k. Progress activity as tolerated
   l. Apply antiembolitic stockings
   m. Monitor VS, UO, I/O, laboratory studies
   n. Monitor and maintain position and patency of drainage tubes: NG, Foley, wound drainage
   o. Encourage ventilation of feelings about change in body image
   p. Monitor and record color, consistency, and amount of stool
   q. Provide routine colostomy care: prevent skin breakdown, assess stoma, control odor, change ostomy bag as needed, irrigate
   r. Increase fluid intake to 3,000 ml/day

4. Possible surgical complications
   a. Infection
   b. Hemorrhage
   c. Dehiscence
   d. Evisceration
   e. Paralytic ileus

     f. Prolapsed stoma

     g. Abscess

  5. Patient/family postoperative teaching goals; the patient will:

     a. Keep follow-up appointments

     b. Maintain regular exercise program

     c. Stop smoking

     d. Maintain ideal weight

     e. State the action, side effects, and scheduling of medications

     f. Recognize the signs and symptoms of infection and intestinal obstruction

     g. Adhere to activity limitations

     h. Complete daily incision care

     i. Use specialized appliances: ostomy bags

     j. Assess condition of stoma daily and report bleeding and changes

     k. Report changes in color and consistency of stools

     l. Perform colostomy care daily

     m. Identify foods that cause flatus and irritability of the colon

     n. Discuss concerns about sexual activities

L. Hiatal hernia (esophageal hernia)

  1. Definition: protrusion of the stomach through the diaphragm into the thoracic cavity

  2. Possible etiology

     a. Congenital weakness

     b. Obesity

     c. Pregnancy

     d. Trauma

     e. Increased abdominal pressure

     f. Aging process

  3. Pathophysiology

     a. The opening (hiatus) in the diaphragm where the esophagus enters the stomach becomes enlarged and weakened

     b. Upper portion of the stomach enters the lower thorax

     c. Sliding of the esophagus and stomach into the chest results in reflux of gastric acid

  4. Possible clinical manifestations

     a. Pyrosis

     b. Dysphagia

     c. Regurgitation

     d. Sternal pain after eating

     e. Vomiting

     f. Feeling of fullness

     g. Dyspnea

     h. Cough

     i. Tachycardia

5. Possible diagnostic test findings
   a. Esophagoscopy: incompetent cardiac sphincter
   b. Barium swallow: protrusion of the hernia
   c. Chest X-ray (CXR): protrusion of abdominal organs into thorax
   d. Gastric analysis: increased pH
6. Medical management
   a. Diet therapy: bland diet with decreased intake of caffeine and spicy foods
   b. Oxygen therapy
   c. GI decompression: NG tube
   d. Position: semi-Fowler
   e. Activity: as tolerated
   f. Monitoring: VS, UO, I/O
   g. Anticholinergics: propantheline bromide (Pro-Banthine)
   h. Antacids: magnesium and aluminum hydroxide (Maalox), aluminum hydroxide gel (Alternagel)
   i. Histamine antagonists: cimetidine (Tagamet), ranitidine (Zantac)
   j. Weight reduction
7. Medical nursing interventions/responsibilities
   a. Maintain diet
   b. Administer oxygen
   c. Assess respiratory status
   d. Maintain position, patency, low suction of NG tube
   e. Maintain semi-Fowler position
   f. Monitor and record VS, UO, I/O, daily weights
   g. Administer medications
   h. Allay anxiety
   i. Avoid flexion at waist in positioning patient
8. Patient/family teaching goals; the patient will:
   a. Keep follow-up appointments
   b. Maintain regular exercise program
   c. Stop smoking
   d. Maintain ideal weight
   e. State the action, side effects, and scheduling of medications
   f. Follow dietary recommendations and restrictions
   g. Eat small, frequent meals
   h. Stop drinking carbonated beverages and alcohol
   i. Maintain upright position for 2 hours after eating
   j. Avoid constrictive clothing
   k. Avoid lifting, bending, straining, coughing
9. Possible medical complications
   a. Hemorrhage
   b. Ulceration
   c. Aspiration
   d. Incarceration of stomach in chest

10. Possible surgical interventions
    a. Reduction of hiatal hernia
    b. Fundoplication

M. Gastric ulcer (peptic ulcer)
   1. Definition: erosion of mucosal lining of stomach
   2. Possible etiology
       a. Alcohol abuse
       b. Stress
       c. Drug-induced: salicylates, steroids, indomethacin, reserpine
       d. Smoking
       e. Gastritis
       f. Zollinger-Ellison syndrome
   3. Pathophysiology
       a. Increased emptying time of gastric acid from the gastric lumen into the gastric mucosa causes an inflammatory reaction with tissue breakdown
       b. Bile refluxes into the stomach if the pyloric valve is involved
       c. Combination of hydrochloric acid and pepsin destroys gastric mucosa
   4. Possible clinical manifestations
       a. Left epigastric pain 1 to 2 hours after eating
       b. Weight loss
       c. Nausea and vomiting
       d. Hematemesis
       e. Melena
       f. Anorexia
       g. Relief of pain after administration of antacids
   5. Possible diagnostic test findings
       a. Hematology: decreased Hgb, Hct
       b. Endoscopy: ulceration
       c. Gastric analysis: normal for gastric ulcer
       d. Upper GI: location of ulcer
       e. Barium swallow: ulceration of gastric mucosa
       f. Stool for occult blood: positive
       g. Serum gastrin: normal or increased
   6. Medical management
       a. Diet therapy: bland
       b. GI decompression: NG tube
       c. Position: semi-Fowler
       d. Activity: bedrest
       e. Monitoring: VS, UO, I/O
       f. Laboratory studies: Hgb, Hct
       g. Treatments: iced saline lavage by NG tube
       h. Transfusion therapy: packed red blood cells (PRBC)
       i. Anticholinergics: propantheline bromide (Pro-Banthine), dicyclomine hydrochloride (Darbid)

     j. Antacids: magnesium and aluminum hydroxide (Maalox), aluminum hydroxide gel (Alternagel)

     k. Histamine antagonists: cimetidine (Tagamet), ranitidine (Zantac)

7. Medical nursing interventions/responsibilities

     a. Maintain diet

     b. Assess respiratory and cardiovascular status

     c. Maintain position, patency, low suction of NG tube

     d. Maintain semi-Fowler position

     e. Monitor and record VS, UO, I/O, laboratory studies, stool for occult blood

     f. Administer medications

     g. Allay anxiety

     h. Provide nares and mouth care

     i. Minimize environmental stress

     j. Maintain a quiet environment

     k. Irrigate NG tube

     l. Monitor consistency, amount, frequency, color of stool

8. Patient/family teaching goals; the patient will:

     a. Keep follow-up appointments

     b. Maintain regular exercise program

     c. Stop smoking

     d. Maintain ideal weight

     e. State the action, side effects, and scheduling of medications

     f. Identify and reduce stress

     g. Follow dietary recommendations and restrictions

     h. Maintain a quiet environment

     i. Avoid caffeine, alcohol, spicy food, fried food

9. Possible medical complications

     a. Hemorrhage

     b. Perforation

     c. Chemical peritonitis

     d. Intestinal obstruction

10. Possible surgical interventions

     a. Bilroth I (see page 119)

     b. Bilroth II (see page 119)

     c. Pyloroplasty and vagotomy (see page 119)

N. Gastric cancer

1. Definition: malignant tumor of the stomach that is primary or metastatic

2. Possible etiology

     a. Increased intake of salted and smoked foods

     b. Dietary deficiency: vegetables, fruits

     c. Chronic gastritis

     d. Achlorhydria

     e. Pernicious anemia

     f. Gastric ulcer

3. Pathophysiology
   a. Unregulated cell growth and uncontrolled cell division result in the development of a neoplasm
   b. Tumor usually develops in distal third of stomach and metastasizes to abdominal organs, lungs, and bones
   c. Most common neoplasm is adenocarcinoma
4. Possible clinical manifestations
   a. Fatigue
   b. Weakness
   c. Syncope
   d. Shortness of breath
   e. Nausea and vomiting
   f. Weight loss
   g. Hematemesis
   h. Indigestion
   i. Epigastric fullness and pain
   j. Malaise
   k. Melena
   l. Regurgitation
   m. Anorexia
5. Possible diagnostic test findings
   a. Stool for occult blood: positive
   b. CEA: positive
   c. Hematology: decreased Hgb, Hct
   d. Blood chemistry: increased SGOT, LDH, amylase
   e. Gastric analysis: positive cancer cells, achlorhydria
   f. GI series: gastric mass
   g. Gastroscopy: biopsy positive for cancer cells
6. Medical management
   a. Diet therapy: high-protein, high-calorie
   b. I.V. therapy: heparin lock
   c. GI decompression: NG tube
   d. Position: semi-Fowler
   e. Activity: as tolerated
   f. Monitoring: VS, UO, I/O
   g. Laboratory studies: Hgb, Hct, stools for occult blood
   h. Nutritional support: IVH
   i. Radiation therapy
   j. Antineoplastics: carmustine (BCNU), 5-fluorouracil (5-FU)
   k. Vitamin supplements: folic acid (Folvite), cyanocobalamin (vitamin B_{12})
   l. Chemotherapy
7. Medical nursing interventions/responsibilities
   a. Maintain diet
   b. Assess GI status
   c. Maintain position, patency, low suction of NG tube

      d. Maintain semi-Fowler position
      e. Monitor and record VS, UO, I/O, laboratory studies, daily weights
      f. Administer IVH
      g. Administer medications
      h. Encourage ventilation of feelings about fear of dying
      i. Provide skin and mouth care
      j. Provide rest periods
      k. Monitor consistency, amount, frequency, and color of stool for blood
      l. Provide postchemotherapeutic and/or postradiation nursing care: provide skin, mouth, and perineal care; encourage dietary intake; administer antiemetics and antidiarrheals; monitor for bleeding, infection, and electrolyte imbalance; provide rest periods

8. Patient/family teaching goals; the patient will:
      a. Keep follow-up appointments
      b. Maintain ideal weight
      c. State the action, side effects, and scheduling of medications
      d. Recognize the signs and symptoms of infection and ulceration
      e. Avoid exposure to people with infections
      f. Alternate rest periods with activity
      g. Monitor self for infection
      h. Follow dietary recommendations and restrictions
      i. Seek help from community agencies and resources
      j. Complete daily skin care

9. Possible medical complications
      a. Obstruction
      b. Ulceration
      c. Metastasis

10. Possible surgical interventions
      a. Subtotal gastrectomy (see page 119)
      b. Total gastrectomy (see page 119)
      c. Bilroth I (see page 119)
      d. Bilroth II (see page 119)

O. Ulcerative colitis

1. Definition: inflammatory disorder of the large bowel
2. Possible etiology
      a. Emotional stress
      b. Autoimmune disease
      c. Genetics
      d. Idiopathic cause
      e. Allergies
      f. Viral and bacterial infections
3. Pathophysiology
      a. Inflammatory edema of the mucous membrane of the colon and rectum leads to bleeding and shallow ulcerations

     b. Abscess formation causes bowel-wall shortening, thinning, fragility, hypermotility, and decreased absorption

     c. Mucosal ulcerations begin in distal end of colon and ascend the large intestine

4. Possible clinical manifestations

     a. Abdominal tenderness

     b. Weakness

     c. Debilitation

     d. Anorexia

     e. Nausea and vomiting

     f. Dehydration

     g. Bloody, purulent, mucoid, watery stools (15 to 20/day)

     h. Elevated temperature

     i. Cachexia

     j. Weight loss

     k. Abdominal cramping

     l. Tenesmus

     m. Hyperactive bowel sounds

     n. Abdominal distention

5. Possible diagnostic test findings

     a. Sigmoidoscopy: ulceration and hyperemia

     b. Barium enema: presence of ulcerations

     c. Blood chemistry: decreased potassium; increased osmolality

     d. Hematology: decreased Hgb, Hct

     e. Urine chemistry: increased specific gravity

     f. Stool specimen: positive for blood and mucus

6. Medical management

     a. Diet therapy: high-protein, high-calorie, low-residue, bland, in small, frequent feedings with restricted intake of milk and gas-forming foods; withhold food and fluids

     b. I.V. therapy: hydration, electrolyte replacement, heparin lock

     c. GI decompession: NG tube

     d. Position: semi-Fowler

     e. Activity: bed rest with bedside commode

     f. Monitoring: VS, UO, I/O, daily weights, specific gravity, calorie count, stool for occult blood

     g. Laboratory studies: potassium, Hgb, Hct, osmolality

     h. Nutritional support: IVH

     i. Treatments: Foley catheter, sitz baths

     j. Antibiotics: sulfasalazine (Azulfidine)

     k. Analgesics: meperidine hydrochloride (Demerol)

     l. Sedatives: phenobarbital (Luminal)

     m. Anticholinergics: propantheline bromide (Pro-Banthine), dicyclomine hydrochloride (Darbid)

     n. Antacids: magnesium and aluminum hydroxide (Maalox), aluminum hydroxide gel (Alternagel)

o. Corticosteroids: hydrocortisone (Solu-Cortef)
p. Antiemetics: prochlorperazine (Compazine)
q. Antidiarrheals: diphenoxylate (Lomotil)
r. Transfusion therapy: PRBC
s. Hematinics: ferrous sulfate (Feosol), ferrous gluconate (Fergon)
t. Immunosuppressive agents: azathioprine (Imuran) cyclophosphamide (Cytoxan)
u. Vitamins and minerals
v. Tranquilizers: diazepam (Valium)
w. Potassium supplement: potassium chloride (K-Lor), potassium gluconate (Kaon)

7. Medical nursing interventions/responsibilities
a. Maintain diet; withhold food and fluids
b. Force tepid fluids
c. Administer I.V. fluids
d. Assess GI status and fluid balance
e. Maintain position, patency, low suction of NG tube
f. Maintain semi-Fowler position
g. Monitor and record VS, UO, I/O, laboratory studies, daily weights, specific gravity, calorie count, stool for occult blood
h. Administer IVH and transfusion therapy
i. Administer medications
j. Allay anxiety
k. Provide skin, mouth, nares, perianal care
l. Maintain bed rest with bedside commode
m. Turn every 2 hours
n. Minimize environmental stress
o. Provide rest periods
p. Maintain a quiet environment
q. Promote independence in activities of daily living (ADL)
r. Assess bowel sounds
s. Administer sitz baths
t. Monitor number, amount, and character of stools
u. Assess perineal excoriation

8. Patient/family teaching goals; the patient will:
a. Keep follow-up appointments
b. Maintain regular exercise program
c. Stop smoking
d. Maintain ideal weight
e. State the action, side effects, and scheduling of medications
f. Identify and reduce stress
g. Recognize the signs and symptoms of rectal hemorrhage and intestinal obstructions
h. Alternate rest periods with activity
i. Follow dietary recommendations and restrictions
j. Maintain a quiet environment

      k. Seek help from community agencies and resources

      l. Complete daily sitz baths and perianal care

9. Possible medical complications

      a. Anemia

      b. Malnutrition

      c. GI perforations

      d. Megacolon

      e. Dehydration

      f. GI obstruction

      g. Hypokalemia

      h. Massive rectal hemorrhage

      i. Amyloidosis

10. Possible surgical interventions

      a. Ileostomy (see page 121)

      b. Colectomy (see page 121)

P. Regional enteritis (Crohn's disease)

1. Definition

      a. Chronic inflammatory disease of the small intestine, usually affecting the terminal ileum and ascending colon

      b. Slowly progressive with exacerbations and remissions

2. Possible etiology

      a. Unknown

      b. Emotional upsets

      c. Milk and milk products

      d. Fried foods

3. Pathophysiology

      a. Ulcerations of intestinal mucosa are accompanied by congestion, thickening of the small bowel, and fissure formations

      b. Enlarged regional mesenteric lymph nodes accompany fibrosis and narrowing of intestinal wall

4. Possible clinical manifestations

      a. Pain in lower right quadrant

      b. Mesenteric lymphadenitis

      c. Abdominal cramps and spasms after meals

      d. Nausea

      e. Flatulence

      f. Weight loss

      g. Elevated temperature

      h. Chronic diarrhea with blood

      i. Borborygmus

5. Possible diagnostic test findings

      a. Abdominal X-ray: congested, thickened, fibrosed, and narrowed intestinal wall

      b. Proctosigmoidoscopy: ulceration

      c. Stool for occult blood: positive

    d. Fecal fat test: increased
    e. Upper GI: classic "string sign" at terminal ileum
    f. Barium enema: lesions in terminal ileum

6. Medical management
    a. Diet therapy: high-protein, high-calorie, low-residue, low-fat, low-fiber, high-carbohydrate, bland, in small, frequent feedings with restricted intake of milk and gas-forming foods; or withhold food and fluids
    b. I.V. therapy: heparin lock
    c. Activity: as tolerated
    d. Monitoring: VS, I/O, daily weights, stool for occult blood, specific gravity
    e. Laboratory studies: potassium, Hgb, Hct, osmolality
    f. Nutritional support: IVH
    g. Antibiotics: sulfasalazine (Azulfidine)
    h. Analgesics: meperidine hydrochloride (Demerol)
    i. Anticholinergics: propantheline bromide (Pro-Banthine), dicyclomine hydrochloride (Darbid)
    j. Antacids: magnesium and aluminum hydroxide (Maalox), aluminum hydroxide gel (Alternagel)
    k. Corticosteroids: prednisone (Deltasone)
    l. Antiemetics: prochlorperazine (Compazine)
    m. Antidiarrheals: diphenoxylate (Lomotil)
    n. Hematinics: ferrous sulfate (Feosol), ferrous gluconate (Fergon)
    o. Vitamins and minerals
    p. Potassium supplement: potassium chloride (K-Lor), potassium gluconate (Kaon)

7. Medical nursing interventions/responsibilities
    a. Maintain diet; withhold food and fluids
    b. Force fluids
    c. Assess GI status and fluid balance
    d. Monitor and record VS, I/O, laboratory studies, daily weights, specific gravity, stool for occult blood
    e. Administer IVH
    f. Administer medications
    g. Allay anxiety
    h. Provide skin and perianal care
    i. Minimize environmental stress
    j. Maintain a quiet environment
    k. Promote independence in ADL
    l. Monitor number, amount, and character of stools
    m. Assess abdominal distention

8. Patient/family teaching goals; the patient will:
    a. Keep follow-up appointments
    b. Maintain regular exercise program
    c. Stop smoking
    d. Maintain ideal weight

      e. State the action, side effects, and scheduling of medications
      f. Identify and reduce stress
      g. Recognize the signs and symptoms of rectal hemorrhage and intestinal obstructions
      h. Alternate rest periods with activity
      i. Follow dietary recommendations and restrictions
      j. Maintain a quiet environment
      k. Seek help from community agencies and resources
      l. Complete daily perianal care
      m. Avoid laxatives and aspirin

9. Possible medical complications
      a. Intestinal obstruction
      b. Intestinal fistulas
      c. Intestinal perforation
      d. Hemorrhage
      e. Malnutrition
      f. Anemia
10. Possible surgical interventions: bowel resection with anastomosis (see page 121)

Q. Diverticulosis/diverticulitis

1. Definition
      a. Diverticulum: outpouching of intestinal mucosa through the muscular wall of the intestine
      b. Diverticulosis: presence of multiple diverticula
      c. Diverticulitis: inflammation of diverticula
2. Possible etiology
      a. Stress
      b. Congenital weakening of intestinal wall
      c. Dietary deficiency: roughage and fiber
      d. Straining at stool
      e. Chronic constipation
3. Pathophysiology
      a. Muscle tone is weakened in the intestinal wall, resulting in a saclike outpouching (diverticulum)
      b. Inflammation (diverculitis) is caused by bacteria and fecal material trapped in the diverticula
      c. Intestinal wall thickens and narrows
      d. Common site is sigmoid colon
4. Possible clinical manifestations
      a. Left lower quadrant pain
      b. Constipation/diarrhea
      c. Bloody stools
      d. Elevated temperature
      e. Rectal bleeding
      f. Change in bowel habits

g. Flatulence
h. Nausea
5. Possible diagnostic test findings
    a. Sigmoidoscopy: diverticula, thickened wall
    b. Barium enema (contraindicated in acute diverticulitis): inflammation, narrow lumen of the bowel, diverticula
    c. Hematology: increased WBC, erythrocyte sedimentation rate (ESR)
6. Medical management
    a. Diet therapy: high-fiber, high-residue
    b. I.V. therapy: hydration, heparin lock
    c. GI decompression: NG tube
    d. Position: semi-Fowler
    e. Activity: bed rest, active ROM, isometric exercises
    f. Monitoring: VS, UO, I/O
    g. Laboratory studies: Hgb, Hct, WBC
    h. Nutritional support: IVH
    i. Antibiotics: gentamicin (Garamycin), tobramycin (Nebcin), clindamycin (Cleocin)
    j. Anticholinergics: propantheline bromide (Pro-Banthine)
    k. Stool softeners: docusate sodium (Colace)
7. Medical nursing interventions/responsibilities
    a. Maintain diet
    b. Assess abdominal distention
    c. Maintain position, patency, low suction of NG tube
    d. Maintain semi-Fowler position
    e. Monitor and record VS, UO, I/O, laboratory studies
    f. Administer IVH
    g. Administer medications
    h. Allay anxiety
    i. Provide nares and mouth care
    j. Provide rest periods
    k. Administer cleansing enemas
    l. Monitor stools for occult blood
    m. Assess bowel sounds
8. Patient/family teaching goals; the patient will:
    a. Keep follow-up appointments
    b. State the action, side effects, and scheduling of medications
    c. Identify and reduce stress
    d. List measures to decrease constipation
    e. Follow dietary recommendations and restrictions
    f. Avoid corn, nuts, fruits, vegetables with seeds
    g. Monitor stools for bleeding
9. Possible medical complications
    a. Bowel perforation
    b. Peritonitis
    c. Abscess

    d. Fistula

    e. Hemorrhage

10. Possible surgical interventions: resection of the bowel (see page 121)

R. Intestinal obstruction

1. Definition: blockage of intestinal lumen
2. Possible etiology
   a. Adhesions
   b. Hernias
   c. Tumors
   d. Fecal impaction
   e. Mesenteric thrombosis
   f. Paralytic ileus
   g. Diverticulitis
   h. Inflammation (Crohn's disease)
   i. Volvulus
3. Pathophysiology
   a. Gas, fluid, and digested substances accumulate proximal to the obstruction
   b. Fluids and gases cause bowel distention
   c. Peristalsis increases proximal to the obstruction
   d. Water and electrolytes are secreted into the blocked bowel
   e. Bowel inflammation increases and absorption by bowel mucosa is inhibited
   f. Fluid loss results in dehydration
4. Possible clinical manifestations
   a. Cramping pain
   b. Nausea
   c. Abdominal distention
   d. Vomiting fecal material
   e. Constipation
   f. Singultus
   g. Elevated temperature
   h. Diminished or absent bowel sounds
   i. Weight loss
5. Possible diagnostic test findings
   a. Blood chemistry: decreased sodium, potassium
   b. Hematology: increased WBC
   c. Barium enema: stops at obstruction
   d. Abdominal X-rays: increased amount of gas in bowel
6. Medical management
   a. Diet therapy: withhold food and fluids
   b. I.V. therapy: hydration, electrolyte replacement; heparin lock
   c. GI decompression: NG tube, Miller-Abbott tube
   d. Position: semi-Fowler
   e. Activity: bed rest

      f. Monitoring: VS, UO, I/O
      g. Laboratory studies: sodium, potassium, WBC
      h. Treatments: Foley catheter, NG irrigation
      i. Antibiotics: gentamicin (Garamycin)
  7. Medical nursing interventions/responsibilities
      a. Withhold food and fluids
      b. Administer I.V. fluids
      c. Assess bowel sounds
      d. Measure abdominal girth
      e. Monitor and record frequency, color, amount of stool
      f. Maintain position, patency, low suction of NG tube and Miller-Abbott tube
      g. Maintain semi-Fowler position
      h. Monitor and record VS, UO, I/O, laboratory studies
      i. Administer medications
      j. Allay anxiety
      k. Provide nares and mouth care
  8. Patient/family teaching goals; the patient will:
      a. Keep follow-up appointments
      b. State the action, side effects, and scheduling of medications
      c. Recognize the signs and symptoms of diverticulitis
      d. Follow dietary recommendations and restrictions
      e. Monitor frequency and color of stool
      f. Avoid constipating foods
  9. Possible medical complications
      a. Peritonitis
      b. Strangulation of bowel
      c. Infection
      d. Sepsis
      e. Bowel necrosis
  10. Possible surgical interventions
      a. Resection of the bowel (see page 121)
      b. Colostomy (see page 121)

S. Peritonitis
  1. Definition: localized or generalized inflammation of peritoneal cavity
  2. Possible etiology
      a. Bacterial infection
      b. Pancreatitis
      c. Blunt or penetrating trauma
      d. Inflammation of colon or kidneys
      e. Volvulus
      f. Intestinal ischemia
      g. Intestinal obstruction
      h. Peptic ulceration
      i. Biliary tract disease

      j. Neoplasms
      k. Nephrosis
      l. Cirrhosis
      m. Intestinal perforation
3. Pathophysiology
      a. Peritoneal irritants cause inflammatory edema, vascular congestion, and hypermotility of the bowel
      b. Movement of extracellular fluid into peritoneal cavity leads to hypovolemia and decreased urine output
4. Possible clinical manifestations
      a. Constant, diffuse, intense abdominal pain
      b. Rebound tenderness
      c. Malaise
      d. Nausea
      e. Elevated temperature
      f. Abdominal rigidity and distention
      g. Anorexia
      h. Decreased urine output
      i. Shallow respirations
      j. Weak, rapid pulse
      k. Decreased peristalsis
      l. Decreased or absent bowel sounds
      m. Abdominal resonance and tympany on percussion
5. Possible diagnostic test findings
      a. Hematology: increased WBC, Hct
      b. Peritoneal aspiration: positive for blood, pus, bile, bacteria, or amylase
      c. Abdominal X-ray: free air in abdomen under diaphragm
6. Medical management
      a. Diet therapy: withhold food or fluid
      b. I.V. therapy: hydration, electrolyte replacement, heparin lock
      c. GI decompression: NG tube
      d. Position: semi-Fowler
      e. Activity: bed rest
      f. Monitoring: VS, UO, I/O, CVP, specific gravity
      g. Laboratory studies: Hgb, Hct, potassium, sodium, calcium, osmolality, WBC
      h. Nutritional support: IVH
      i. Treatments: Foley catheter, incentive spirometry
      j. Antibiotics: gentamicin (Garamycin), clindamycin (Cleocin), cephalothin (Keflin)
      k. Analgesics: meperidine hydrochloride (Demerol)
7. Medical nursing interventions/responsibilities
      a. Withhold food and fluids
      b. Administer I.V. fluids
      c. Provide pulmonary toilet: TCDB
      d. Assess respiratory status and fluid balance

  e. Maintain position, patency, low suction of NG tube
  f. Maintain semi-Fowler position
  g. Monitor and record VS, UO, I/O, laboratory studies, CVP, daily weights, specific gravity
  h. Administer IVH
  i. Administer medications
  j. Allay anxiety
  k. Provide nares and mouth care
  l. Turn every 2 hours
  m. Maintain bed rest
  n. Assess pain
  o. Assess bowel sounds
  p. Measure abdominal girth
  q. Avoid use of laxatives
  r. Do not apply heat to abdomen
 8. Patient/family teaching goals; the patient will:
  a. Keep follow-up appointments
  b. State the action, side effects, and scheduling of medications
  c. Recognize the signs and symptoms of GI obstruction
  d. Follow dietary recommendations and restrictions
 9. Possible medical complications
  a. Adhesions
  b. Abscesses
  c. Obstructions
  d. Septic shock
  e. Paralytic ileus
10. Possible surgical interventions
  a. Exploratory laparotomy
  b. Bowel resection (see page 121)
  c. Incision and drainage of abscess
  d. Closure of perforation

T. Hemorrhoids
 1. Definition: congested and dilated internal or external vessels of the rectum and anus
 2. Possible etiology
  a. Chronic constipation
  b. Prolonged sitting or standing
  c. Straining at stool
  d. Pregnancy
  e. Heavy lifting
  f. Portal hypertension
  g. Heredity
  h. Obesity
  i. Anal infection

3. Pathophysiology
   a. Increased abdominal pressure impairs the flow of blood through the hemorrhoidal venous plexus
   b. Decreased blood flow causes dilation and congestion of the vessels of the rectum and anus
4. Possible clinical manifestations
   a. Anal pain with defecation, sitting, or walking
   b. Anal pruritus
   c. Protrusion of hemorrhoids
   d. Rectal bleeding
   e. Rectal mucous discharge
   f. Bleeding during defecation
   g. Sensation of incomplete fecal evacuation
5. Possible diagnostic test findings
   a. Digital exam: presence of hemorrhoids
   b. Barium enema: prescence of hemorrhoids
   c. Proctoscopy: presence of internal hemorrhoids
   d. Hematology: decreased Hgb, Hct
6. Medical management
   a. Diet therapy: high-fiber, low-roughage, with increased fluid intake
   b. Position: side-lying or prone
   c. Activity: as tolerated
   d. Monitoring: VS, frequency of stools
   e. Laboratory studies: Hgb, Hct
   f. Treatments: witch hazel compresses, sitz baths
   g. Corticosteroids: hydrocortisone (Hydrocortisone cream)
   h. Analgesics: acetaminophen (Tylenol)
   i. Antipruritics: diphenhydramine (Benadryl)
   j. Stool softeners: docusate sodium (Colace)
   k. Anesthetics: lidocaine hydrochloride (Xylocaine)
   l. Laxative: magnesium hydroxide (Milk of Magnesia)
   m. Cryodestruction
7. Medical nursing interventions/responsibilities
   a. Maintain diet with increased fluids
   b. Assess bowel elimination and rectal bleeding
   c. Maintain side-lying or prone position
   d. Monitor and record VS, I/O, laboratory studies
   e. Administer medications
   f. Allay anxiety
   g. Provide perineal care
   h. Administer sitz baths and witch hazel compresses
   i. Provide privacy and time for defecation
8. Patient/family teaching goals; the patient will:
   a. Keep follow-up appointments
   b. Maintain regular exercise program
   c. Maintain ideal weight

    d. State the action, side effects, and scheduling of medications
    e. Recognize the signs and symptoms of rectal bleeding
    f. Avoid heavy lifting, prolonged sitting or standing
    g. Follow dietary recommendations and restrictions
    h. Complete daily perineal care
    i. Avoid constipation
    j. Defecate when urge is felt
    k. Use sitz baths and witch hazel compresses
9. Possible medical complications
    a. Megacolon
    b. Diverticulitis
    c. Hemorrhage
10. Possible surgical interventions
    a. Hemorrhoidectomy (see page 120)
    b. Barron rubber-band ligation

U. Colorectal cancer

1. Definition: malignant tumor of the colon or rectum that is primary or metastatic
2. Possible etiology
    a. Diverticulosis
    b. Chronic ulcerative colitis
    c. Familial polyposis
    d. Aging process
    e. Low-fiber, high-carbohydrate diet
    f. Chronic constipation
3. Pathophysiology
    a. Unregulated cell growth and uncontrolled cell division result in the development of a neoplasm
    b. Metastasis often occurs in the liver
    c. Adenocarcinomas occur in the colon, rectum, jejunum, and duodenum
    d. Adenocarcinomas infiltrate and cause obstruction, ulcerations, and hemorrhage
4. Possible clinical manifestations
    a. Abdominal cramps
    b. Abdominal distention
    c. Diarrhea/constipation
    d. Weakness
    e. Pallor
    f. Weight loss
    g. Anorexia
    h. Change in shape of stool
    i. Rectal bleeding
    j. Palpable mass
    k. Fecal oozing
    l. Change in bowel habits

m. Melena

n. Vomiting

5. Possible diagnostic test findings
   a. Stool for occult blood: positive
   b. Hematology: decreased Hgb, Hct
   c. Sigmoidoscopy: identification and location of mass
   d. Barium enema: location of mass
   e. Biopsy: cytology positive for cancer cells
   f. CEA: positive
   g. GI series: location of mass

6. Medical management
   a. Diet therapy: High-fiber, low-fat, low-refined carbohydrate diet
   b. I.V. therapy: heparin lock
   c. Position: semi-Fowler
   d. Activity: as tolerated
   e. Monitoring: VS, U/O, I/O
   f. Laboratory studies: Hgb, Hct
   g. Nutritional support: IVH
   h. Radiation therapy
   i. Antineoplastics: doxorubicin hydrochloride (Adriamycin), 5-fluorouracil (5-FU)
   j. Chemotherapy

7. Medical nursing interventions/responsibilities
   a. Maintain diet
   b. Maintain semi-Fowler position
   c. Monitor and record VS, UO, I/O, laboratory studies, daily weights
   d. Administer IVH
   e. Administer medications
   f. Encourage ventilation of feelings about change in body image and fear of dying
   g. Provide skin and mouth care
   h. Provide rest periods
   i. Monitor and record color, consistency, amount, and frequency of stool
   j. Assess for signs of intestinal obstruction and rectal bleeding
   k. Provide postchemotherapeutic and/or postradiation nursing care: provide skin, mouth, and perineal care; encourage dietary intake; administer antiemetics and antidiarrheals; monitor for bleeding, infection, and electrolyte imbalance; provide rest periods

8. Patient/family teaching goals; the patient will:
   a. Keep follow-up appointments
   b. Maintain ideal weight
   c. State the action, side effects, and scheduling of medications
   d. Recognize the signs and symptoms of infection
   e. Alternate rest periods with activity
   f. Monitor self for infection
   g. Follow dietary recommendations and restrictions

  h. Seek help from community agencies and resources
  i. Monitor changes in bowel elimination
9. Possible medical complications
  a. Anemia
  b. Hemorrhage
  c. Intestinal obstruction
10. Possible surgical interventions
  a. Abdominoperineal resection (see page 121)
  b. Colostomy (see page 121)

V. Cholecystitis
1. Definition: acute or chronic inflammation of the gall bladder; most commonly associated with cholelithiasis
2. Possible etiology
  a. Cholelithiasis: cholesterol, bile pigment, calcium stones
  b. Obesity
  c. Infection of the gall bladder
  d. Estrogen therapy
3. Pathophysiology
  a. Inflammed gall bladder cannot contract in response to fatty foods entering the duodenum because of obstruction by calculi or edema
  b. Inability to constrict causes pain
  c. Accumulated bile is absorbed into the blood
4. Possible clinical manifestations
  a. Indigestion or chest pain after eating fatty or fried foods
  b. Episodic colicky pain in epigastric area, which radiates to back and shoulder
  c. Nausea and vomiting
  d. Elevated temperature
  e. Jaundice
  f. Flatulence
  g. Belching
  h. Clay-colored stools
  i. Dark amber urine
  j. Pruritus
  k. Ecchymosis
  l. Steatorrhea
5. Possible diagnostic test findings
  a. Cholangiogram: stones in biliary tree
  b. Gall bladder series: stones in biliary tree
  c. Ultrasound: bile duct distention and calculi
  d. Liver scan: obstruction of biliary tree
  e. Blood chemistry: increased alkaline phosphatase, bilirubin, direct bilirubin transaminase, amylase, lipase
  f. Hematology: increased WBC

6. Medical management
   a. Diet therapy: low-fat, high-carbohydrate, high-protein, low-calorie, in small, frequent feedings with restricted intake of gas-forming foods; withhold food and fluids as ordered
   b. I.V. therapy: hydration, electrolyte replacement; heparin lock
   c. GI decompression: NG tube, Miller-Abbott tube
   d. Position: semi-Fowler
   e. Activity: bed rest
   f. Monitoring: VS, U/O, I/O, specific gravity
   g. Laboratory studies: amylase, lipase, bilirubin, alkaline phosphatase, WBC
   h. Treatments: incentive spirometry, tepid baths without soap
   i. Antilithics: chenodiol (Chenix)
   j. Antibiotics: cephalothin (Keflin)
   k. Analgesics: meperidine hydrochloride (Demerol)
   l. Anticholinergics: propantheline bromide (Pro-Banthine), dicyclomine hydrochloride (Darbid)
   m. Antiemetics: prochlorperazine (Compazine)
   n. Antipruritics: diphenhydramine hydrochloride (Benadryl)
   o. Vitamins: phytonadione (AquaMEPHYTON), cyanocobalamine (vitamin B_{12})
7. Medical nursing interventions/responsibilities
   a. Maintain diet; withhold food and fluids
   b. Administer I.V. fluids
   c. Provide pulmonary toilet: TCDB
   d. Assess pain
   e. Maintain position, patency, low suction of NG tube
   f. Maintain semi-Fowler position
   g. Monitor and record VS, U/O, I/O, laboratory studies, specific gravity
   h. Administer medications
   i. Allay anxiety
   j. Provide skin, nares, and mouth care
   k. Maintain bed rest
   l. Maintain a quiet environment
   m. Administer tepid baths without soap
   n. Prevent scratching
8. Patient/family teaching goals; the patient will:
   a. Keep follow-up appointments
   b. Maintain regular exercise program
   c. Stop smoking
   d. Maintain ideal weight
   e. State the action, side effects, and scheduling of medications
   f. Recognize the signs and symptoms of renal colic
   g. Follow dietary recommendations and restrictions
   h. Complete daily skin care

9. Possible medical complications
   a. Hemorrhage
   b. Cirrhosis
   c. Intestinal perforation
   d. Peritonitis
   e. Pancreatitis
10. Possible surgical interventions
   a. Cholecystectomy (see page 116)
   b. Choledochostomy (see page 116)
   c. Cholecystostomy (see page 116)

W. Pancreatitis

1. Definition: acute or chronic inflammation of the pancreas with varying degrees of pancreatic edema, fat necrosis, and hemorrhage
2. Possible etiology
   a. Biliary tract disease
   b. Alcoholism
   c. Hyperparathyroidism
   d. Hyperlipidemia
   e. Blunt trauma to pancreas or abdomen
   f. Bacterial or viral infection
   g. Duodenal ulcer
   h. Drug induced: steroids, thiazide diuretics, oral contraceptives
3. Pathophysiology
   a. Acute: pancreatic enzymes are activated in the pancreas rather than the duodenum, resulting in tissue damage and autodigestion of the pancreas
   b. Chronic: chronic inflammation results in fibrosis and calcification of the pancreas, obstruction of the ducts, and destruction of the secreting acinar cells
4. Possible clinical manifestations
   a. Nausea and vomiting
   b. Tachycardia
   c. Abrupt onset of pain in epigastric area that radiates to the shoulder, substernal area, back, and flank
   d. Aching, burning, stabbing, pressing pain
   e. Abdominal tenderness and distention
   f. Elevated temperature
   g. Steatorrhea
   h. Weight loss
   i. Jaundice
   j. Hypotension
   k. Pain upon eating
   l. Dyspnea
   m. Decreased or absent bowel sounds

5. Possible diagnostic test findings
   a. CT scan: enlarged pancreas
   b. Blood chemistry: increased amylase, lipase, glucose, lipids; decreased calcium, potassium
   c. Hematology: increased WBC
   d. Grey Turner's sign: positive
   e. Ultrasonography: presence of cysts
   f. Cullen's sign: positive
   g. Urine chemistry: increased amylase
   h. Stool for fecal fat: positive
   i. Arteriography: fibrous tissue and calcification of pancreas
   j. Glucose tolerance test: increased
6. Medical management
   a. Diet therapy: low-fat, low-protein, high-carbohydrate, in small, frequent feedings with restricted intake of caffeine, alcohol, and gas-forming foods
   b. I.V. therapy: hydration, electrolyte replacement; heparin lock
   c. GI decompression: NG tube
   d. Position: semi-Fowler
   e. Activity: bed rest
   f. Monitoring: VS, UO, I/O, CVP, specific gravity, urine glucose and ketones
   g. Laboratory studies: glucose, potassium, amylase, lipase, calcium, lipids
   h. Nutritional support: IVH
   i. Transfusion therapy: PRBC
   j. Antibiotics: cephalothin (Keflin)
   k. Analgesics: meperidine hydrochloride (Demerol)
   l. Anticholinergics: propantheline bromide (Pro-Banthine), dicyclomine hydrochloride (Darbid)
   m. Antacids: magnesium and aluminum hydroxide (Maalox), aluminum hydroxide gel (Alternagel)
   n. Corticosteroids: hydrocortisone (Solu-Cortef)
   o. Antiemetics: prochlorperazine (Compazine)
   p. Histamine antagonists: cimetidine (Tagamet), ranitidine (Zantac)
   q. Vitamins and minerals
   r. Tranquilizers: diazepam (Valium)
   s. Hormones: pancreatin (Viokase), lipase (Cotazym)
   t. Potassium supplement: potassium chloride (K-Lor), potassium gluconate (Kaon)
   u. Peritoneal lavage
   v. Dialysis
   w. Calcium supplement: calcium gluconate (Kalcinate), calcium carbonate (Os-Cal)
   x. Antidiabetic agent: insulin

7. Medical nursing interventions/responsibilities
   a. Maintain diet; withhold food and fluids
   b. Administer I.V. fluids
   c. Assess fluid balance
   d. Maintain position, patency, low suction of NG tube
   e. Maintain semi-Fowler position
   f. Monitor and record VS, UO, I/O, laboratory studies, CVP, daily weights, specific gravity, urine glucose and ketones
   g. Administer IVH
   h. Administer medications
   i. Allay anxiety
   j. Provide skin, nares, and mouth care
   k. Maintain bed rest and turn every 2 hours
   l. Provide a quiet, restful environment
   m. Monitor urine and stool for color, character, and amount
8. Patient/family teaching goals; the patient will:
   a. Keep follow-up appointments
   b. Stop smoking
   c. Maintain ideal weight
   d. State the action, side effects, and scheduling of medications
   e. Recognize the signs and symptoms of infection and increased blood sugar
   f. Adhere to activity limitations
   g. Alternate rest periods with activity
   h. Monitor self for infection
   i. Follow dietary recommendations and restrictions
   j. Maintain a quiet environment
   k. Monitor self for steatorrhea
   l. Monitor urine for glucose and ketones
9. Possible medical complications
   a. Ileus
   b. Hypovolemic shock
   c. Diabetes mellitus
   d. Infection
   e. Jaundice
   f. Pancreatic fistula
   g. Pancreatic abscess
10. Possible surgical interventions: pancreatectomy (see page 116)

X. Hepatic cirrhosis
1. Definition
   a. Chronic, progressive disease characterized by inflammation, fibrosis, and degeneration of liver parenchymal cells
   b. Types: Laennec's (micronodular); postnecrotic (macronodular); biliary

2. Possible etiology
   a. Alcohol use or abuse
   b. Malnutrition
   c. Viral hepatitis
   d. Cholecystitis
3. Pathophysiology
   a. Inflammation causes liver parenchymal cell destruction, with subsequent fibrosis
   b. Fibrotic changes cause obstruction of hepatic blood flow and normal liver function
   c. Obstruction causes portal hypertension
   d. Decreased liver function results in decreased absorption and utilization of fat-soluble vitamins (A, D, E, K), increased secretion of aldosterone, and ineffective detoxification of protein wastes
4. Possible clinical manifestations
   a. Nausea and vomiting
   b. Weakness and fatigue
   c. Anorexia and weight loss
   d. Jaundice
   e. Ecchymosis
   f. Palmar erythema
   g. Indigestion
   h. Pruritus
   i. Irregular bowel habits
   j. Pain in right upper quadrant
   k. Peripheral edema
   l. Petechiae
   m. Epistaxis
   n. Hematemesis
   o. Telangiectasis
   p. Gynecomastia and impotence
   q. Amenorrhea
   r. Hemorrhoids
   s. Hepatomegaly
5. Possible diagnostic test findings
   a. Blood chemistry: increased SGOT, SGPT, LDH, alkaline phosphatase, ammonia, bilirubin, BSP; decreased albumin
   b. Hematology: decreased Hgb, Hct, WBC; increased PT
   c. Liver scan: fibrotic liver, increased uptake
   d. Liver biopsy: destruction of parenchymal cells
   e. Esophagoscopy: presence of esophageal varices
   f. Arterial blood gases (ABGs): metabolic acidosis
   g. Urine chemistry: proteinuria

6. Medical management
   a. Diet therapy: high-calorie, high-carbohydrate, low-fat, low-sodium, in small, frequent feedings with restricted intake of alcohol, fluids, and protein
   b. I.V. therapy: hydration, electrolyte replacement; heparin lock
   c. Oxygen therapy
   d. GI decompression: NG tube, Sengsten-Blakemore tube
   e. Position: semi-Fowler
   f. Activity: bed rest
   g. Monitoring: VS, U/O, I/O, neurovital signs, EKG, hemodynamic variables, stools for occult blood
   h. Laboratory studies: SGOT, SGPT, LDH, PT, amylase, lipase, Hgb, Hct, bilirubin, albumin, WBC, ABGs
   i. Nutritional support: IVH, NG feedings
   j. Treatments: Foley catheter, incentive spirometry, tepid bath, cool, moist compresses
   k. Precautions: enteric and protective
   l. Transfusion therapy: platelets, PRBC, fresh frozen plasma (FFP)
   m. Antibiotics: neomycin sulfate (Neobiotic)
   n. Diuretics: spironolactone (Aldactone), furosemide (Lasix)
   o. Sedatives: phenobarbital (Luminal)
   p. Stool softeners: docusate sodium (Colace)
   q. Ammonia detoxicant: lactulose (Cephulac)
   r. Vitamins: phytonadione (AquaMEPHYTON), cyanocobalamine (vitamin B_{12})
   s. Antacids: magnesium and aluminum hydroxide (Maalox), aluminum hydroxide gel (Alternagel)
   t. Analgesics: oxycodone hydrochloride (Tylox)
   u. Enzyme replacement: pancreatin (Viokase)
7. Medical nursing interventions/responsibilities
   a. Maintain diet; withhold food and fluids
   b. Administer I.V. fluids
   c. Administer oxygen
   d. Provide pulmonary toilet: TCDB, incentive spirometry
   e. Assess respiratory status, GI bleeding, and fluid balance
   f. Maintain position, patency, low suction of NG tube
   g. Maintain semi-Fowler position
   h. Monitor and record VS, UO, I/O, laboratory studies, hemodynamic variables, daily weights, specific gravity, stool for occult blood, neurovital signs
   i. Measure abdominal girth
   j. Monitor for infection
   k. Administer IVH
   l. Administer medications
   m. Allay anxiety
   n. Provide skin, mouth, and nares care

     o. Maintain enteric and protective precautions
     p. Maintain bed rest
     q. Maintain a quiet environment
     r. Administer tepid baths without soap; cool, moist compresses
     s. Prevent scratching
     t. Use small-gauge needle for intramuscular injections
     u. Apply prolonged pressure after venipuncture
     v. Monitor stool for color, consistency, and amount
8. Patient/family teaching goals; the patient will:
     a. Keep follow-up appointments
     b. Stop smoking
     c. Maintain ideal weight
     d. State the action, side effects, and scheduling of medications
     e. Avoid use of alcohol
     f. Recognize the signs and symptoms of GI bleeding
     g. Avoid exposure to people with infections
     h. Alternate rest periods with activity
     i. Monitor self for infection
     j. Follow dietary recommendations and restrictions
     k. Complete daily skin care
     l. Avoid straining at stool, vigorous blowing of nose, coughing, and use of hard toothbrush
     m. Avoid use of over-the-counter medications
9. Possible medical complications
     a. Ascites
     b. Esophageal varices
     c. Hemorrhoids
     d. Hemorrhage
     e. Estrogen/androgen imbalance
     f. Portal hypertension
     g. Hepatic coma
     h. Pancytopenia
10. Possible surgical interventions
     a. Portacaval shunt (see page 117)
     b. LeVeen peritoneovenous shunt

Y. Hepatitis
1. Definition
     a. Inflammation of the liver
     b. Types: hepatitis A (infectious); hepatitis B (serum); non-A, non-B hepatitis
2. Possible etiology
     a. Contaminated food, milk, water (hepatitis A)
     b. Contaminated needles (hepatitis A, hepatitis B)
     c. RNA virus (hepatitis A)
     d. DNA virus (hepatitis B)

   e. Blood transfusions (non-A, non-B hepatitis)
   f. Blood, saliva, semen (hepatitis B)
3. Pathophysiology
   a. Inflammation of liver tissue causes inflammation of hepatic cells,
       hypertrophy, and proliferation of Kupffer cells and bile stasis
   b. Type A virus (HAV) is transmitted by fecal or oral route and causes
       hepatitis A
   c. Type B virus (HBV) is transmitted by blood and body fluids and causes
       hepatitis B
4. Possible clinical manifestations
   a. Preicteric: anorexia, nausea, vomiting, fatigue, constipation/diarrhea,
       weight loss, right upper quadrant pain, hepatomegaly, splenomegaly,
       malaise, elevated temperature, pharyngitis, nasal discharge, headache,
       pruritus
   b. Icteric: fatigue, weight loss, clay-colored stools, dark urine,
       hepatomegaly, jaundice, splenomegaly, pruritus
   c. Posticteric: fatigue, decreasing hepatomegaly, decreasing jaundice,
       improved appetite
5. Possible diagnostic test findings
   a. Blood chemistry: increased SGPT, SGOT, alkaline phosphatase, LDH,
       bilirubin, ESR, positive anti-HAV (IgM) or positive HBsAg (surface
       antigen)
   b. Hematology: increased PT
   c. BSP: increased
   d. Urine chemistry: increased urobilinogen
   e. Stool: hepatitis A virus
6. Medical management
   a. Diet therapy: high-calorie, moderate-protein, low-fat
   b. Activity: bed rest
   c. Monitoring: VS, UO, I/O
   d. Laboratory studies: SGPT, SGOT, LDH, bilirubin, PT, PTT
   e. Precautions: enteric (hepatitis A); body/fluid (hepatitis B and non-A,
       non-B)
   f. Antiemetics: prochlorperazine (Compazine)
   g. Vitamins and minerals: vitamin K (AquaMEPHYTON)
7. Medical nursing interventions/responsibilities
   a. Maintain diet
   b. Monitor and record VS, UO, I/O, laboratory studies
   c. Administer medications
   d. Allay anxiety
   e. Maintain body fluid and enteric precautions
   f. Provide rest periods
   g. Encourage small, frequent meals
8. Patient/family teaching goals; the patient will:
   a. Keep follow-up appointments
   b. State the action, side effects, and scheduling of medications

    c. Avoid exposure to people with infections
    d. Alternate rest periods with activity
    e. Monitor self for infection
    f. Follow dietary recommendations and restrictions
    g. Avoid alcohol
    h. Maintain good personal hygiene
    i. Refrain from donating blood
    j. Increase fluid intake to 3,000 ml/day
    k. Abstain from sexual intercourse until serum liver studies are within normal limits

9. Possible medical complications
    a. Pancreatitis
    b. Aplastic anemia
    c. Glomerulonephritis
    d. Vasculitis

10. Possible surgical interventions: none

Z. Esophageal varices

1. Definition: dilation of esophageal veins in the lower part of the esophagus
2. Possible etiology
    a. Portal hypertension
    b. Increased intra-abdominal pressure
    c. Alcohol abuse
    d. Cirrhosis
3. Pathophysiology
    a. Venous drainage from the liver into the portal vein is decreased
    b. Drainage obstruction results in portal hypertension
    c. Return of venous blood from the intestinal tract and spleen to the right atrium via the collateral circulation is obstructed
    d. The increased pressure dilates the esophageal veins, which then protrude into the esophageal lumen
4. Possible clinical manifestations
    a. Anorexia
    b. Nausea and vomiting
    c. Hematemesis
    d. Fatigue and weakness
    e. Splenomegaly
    f. Ascites
    g. Peripheral edema
    h. Melena
    i. Dysphagia
    j. Pallor
5. Possible diagnostic test findings
    a. Hematology: increased PT; decreased RBC, Hgb, Hct
    b. Blood chemistry: increased BUN, LDH, SGOT; decreased albumin

      c. Barium swallow: narrowed and irregular esophagus
      d. Esophagoscopy: varices
6. Medical management
      a. Diet therapy: withhold food and fluids
      b. I.V. therapy: hydration; heparin lock
      c. Oxygen therapy
      d. GI decompression: NG tube
      e. Position: semi-Fowler
      f. Activity: bed rest
      g. Monitoring: VS, UO, I/O
      h. Laboratory studies: Hgb, Hct, PT, PTT
      i. Treatments: Foley catheter
      j. Transfusion therapy: PRBC
      k. Sengstaken-Blakemore tube
      l. Paracentesis
      m. Injection sclerotherapy: 5% morrhuate sodium
      n. Diuretics: furosemide (Lasix)
      o. Hormones: vasopressin tannate (Pitressin)
      p. Antacids: magnesium and aluminum hydroxide (Maalox), aluminum hydroxide gel (Alternagel)
      q. Histamine antagonists: cimetidine (Tagamet), ranitidine (Zantac)
      r. Vitamins: vitamin K (AquaMEPHYTON)
      s. Iced saline lavage by NG tube
      t. Stool softeners: docusate sodium (Colace)
7. Medical nursing interventions/responsibilities
      a. Withhold food and fluids
      b. Administer I.V. fluids
      c. Administer oxygen
      d. Assess cardiovascular and respiratory status
      e. Maintain position, patency, low suction of NG tube and Sengstaken-Blakemore tube
      f. Maintain semi-Fowler position
      g. Monitor and record VS, UO, I/O, laboratory studies, CVP, daily weights
      h. Administer medications
      i. Allay anxiety
      j. Provide nares and mouth care
      k. Minimize environmental stress
      l. Assess for signs of bleeding
      m. Avoid activities that increase intra-abdominal pressure
      n. Monitor amount, color, frequency, and consistency of stools
      o. Assess level of consciousness
8. Patient/family teaching goals; the patient will:
      a. Keep follow-up appointments
      b. Stop smoking
      c. State the action, side effects, and scheduling of medications

      d. Identify and reduce stress
      e. Monitor stools for occult blood
      f. Avoid lifting and straining
      g. Follow dietary recommendations and restrictions
      h. Avoid use of alcohol

9. Possible medical complications
      a. Hemorrhage
      b. Shock
      c. Metabolic imbalance

10. Possible surgical interventions
      a. Ligation of varices
      b. Portacaval shunt (see page 117)
      c. Splenorenal shunt (see page 117)
      d. Mesocaval shunt (see page 117)

Points to Remember

Occult blood in stool and emesis is a common finding in gastrointestinal disorders.

Modifications in dietary habits and life-style are necessary to alter the progression of gastrointestinal illness.

Patients with gastrointestinal disorders should be assessed frequently for dehydration, hyponatremia, and hypokalemia.

Imposed changes in eating and bowel habits may result in social isolation.

Intestinal obstruction and peritonitis are potential complications of all abdominal surgical procedures.

Glossary

Ascites — presence of fluid in the peritoneal cavity.

Dysphagia — difficulty in swallowing.

Hematemesis — vomiting of blood.

Melena — black, tarry stools.

Steatorrhea — fatty stools.

Endocrine System

Learning Objectives

After studying this section, the reader should be able to:

- Describe the psychosocial impact of endocrine system disorders.

- Differentiate between modifiable and nonmodifiable risk factors in the development of an endocrine system disorder.

- List three potential and three actual nursing diagnoses for the patient with an endocrine system disorder.

- Identify the medical and surgical nursing interventions/responsibilities for the patient with an endocrine system disorder.

- Write three teaching goals for the patient with an endocrine system disorder.

V. Endocrine System

A. **Anatomy and physiology**
   1. Hypothalamus
      a. Controls temperature, respiration, and blood pressure
      b. Affects emotional states: fear, anxiety, anger, rage, pleasure, and pain
      c. Produces hypothalamic-stimulating hormones, which affect the inhibition and release of pituitary hormones
   2. Pituitary gland
      a. This "master gland" is composed of anterior and posterior lobes
      b. Posterior lobe (neurohypophysis) secretes vasopressin (antidiuretic hormone: ADH) and oxytocin
      c. Anterior lobe (adenohypophysis) secretes follicle-stimulating hormone (FSH), luteinizing hormone (LH), prolactin, adrenocorticotropic hormone (ACTH), thyroid-stimulating hormone (TSH), and growth hormone (GH)
   3. Thyroid gland
      a. Accelerates cellular reactions, including basal metabolic rate (BMR) and growth
      b. Controlled by secretion of TSH
      c. Produces thyroxin (T4), tri-iodothyronine (T3), and thyrocalcitonin
   4. Parathyroid glands
      a. Secrete parathyroid hormone (parathormone; PTH), which regulates calcium and phosphorus metabolism
      b. Require active form of vitamin D for PTH function
   5. Adrenal glands
      a. Adrenal cortex secretes three major hormones: glucocorticoids (cortisol), mineralocorticoids (aldosterone), and sex hormones (androgens, estrogens, and progesterone)
      b. Adrenal medulla secretes norepinephrine and epinephrine
   6. Pancreas
      a. Accessory gland of digestion
      b. Exocrine function: secretion of digestive enzymes (amylase, lipase, and trypsin)
      c. Endocrine funcion: secretion of insulin, glucagon, somatostatin, and hormones (gastrin, secretin, cholecystokinin, and gastric inhibitory peptide) from islets of Langerhans
      d. Main pancreatic duct joins the common bile duct and empties into the duodenum at the ampulla of Vater

B. **Physical assessment findings**
   1. Subjective data that often accompany endocrine disorders
      a. Change in weight
      b. Change in hair quality and distribution
      c. Change in body proportions, muscle mass, and fat distribution
      d. Fatigue and weakness

      e. Change in mood or behavior

      f. Change in eating patterns: anorexia

      g. Change in bowel habits: constipation, diarrhea

      h. Urinary frequency

      i. Change in menses and libido

      j. History of infections

      k. Intolerance of heat or cold

  2. Objective data to evaluate in endocrine disorders

      a. Vital signs (VS)

      b. Skin color and temperature

      c. Change in level of consciousness

      d. Pattern and character of respirations

      e. Change in urinary patterns

      f. Change in thirst

      g. Abnormalities of nails

      h. Change in visual acuity

C. Diagnostic tests and procedures used to evaluate endocrine disorders

  1. Venous sampling

      a. Definition/purpose: assessment of serial hormone levels after insertion of a catheter

      b. Nursing interventions/responsibilities: before procedure, withhold food and fluids; after procedure, assess for bleeding at insertion site

  2. Hematologic studies

      a. Definition/purpose: laboratory analysis of blood sample for white blood cells (WBC), red blood cells (RBC), erythrocyte sedimentation rate (ESR), platelets, prothrombin time (PT), partial thromboplastin time (PTT), hemoglobin (Hgb), and hematocrit (Hct)

      b. Nursing interventions/responsibilities: assess insertion site for bleeding; note current drug therapy

  3. Blood chemistry

      a. Definition/purpose: laboratory analysis of blood sample for potassium, sodium, calcium, phosphorus, ketones, glucose, osmolality, chloride, blood urea nitrogen (BUN), creatinine (Cr), T3, T4, protein-bound iodine (PBI), cortisol

      b. Nursing interventions/responsibilities: before procedure, withhold food and fluids as ordered; note previous studies using radiopaque dyes; note pregnancy; note drugs being taken that contain iodine; after procedure, assess site for bleeding

  4. Fasting serum glucose and two-hour postprandial glucose test

      a. Definition/purpose: laboratory analysis of blood sample to measure the body's use and disposal of glucose

      b. Nursing interventions/responsibilities: withhold food and fluids for 8 hours before fasting sample is drawn; withhold insulin; give 100 grams of glucose orally and request laboratory to draw blood 2 hours later; assess patient for hypoglycemia or hyperglycemia

5. Glucose tolerance test (GTT)
   a. Definition/purpose: laboratory analysis of blood and urine to measure absorption of carbohydrates
   b. Nursing interventions/responsibilities: note drugs that may interfere with test; note pregnancy, trauma, or infectious disease; give patient high-carbohydrate diet 2 days before test, then have patient fast 12 hours before test begins; instruct patient to avoid smoking, coffee, alcohol, and exercise for 8 hours before procedure; withhold all medications; obtain fasting serum glucose and urine specimen; administer test load oral glucose and record time; request laboratory collection of serum glucose and urine specimens at 30, 60, 120, and 180 minutes; refrigerate samples; assess patient for hyperglycemia or hypoglycemia
6. Adrenocorticotropic hormone (ACTH) stimulation test
   a. Definition/purpose: laboratory analysis of blood sample for cortisol
   b. Nursing interventions/responsibilities: note drugs that may interfere with test; monitor 24-hour I.V. infusion of ACTH after baseline serum sample is drawn; after procedure, assess site for bleeding
7. Dexamethasone suppression test
   a. Definition/purpose: laboratory analysis of serum cortisol and urinary 17-hydroxycorticosteroids after administration of dexamethasone
   b. Nursing interventions/responsibilities; administer dexamethasone and an antacid as ordered; obtain single urine and 24-hour urine samples as ordered; note drugs that might interfere with test
8. 24-hour urine test for 17-ketosteroids (17-KS) and 17-hydroxycorticosteroids (17-OHCS)
   a. Definition/purpose: quantitative laboratory analysis of urine collected over 24 hours to determine hormone precursors
   b. Nursing interventions/responsibilities: withhold all medications for 48 hours before test; instruct patient to void and note time (collection of urine starts with the next voiding); place urine container on ice; measure each voided urine; instruct patient to void at end of 24-hour period; note medications that might interfere with test
9. Urine vanillylmandelic acid test (VMA)
   a. Definition/purpose: quantitative laboratory analysis of urine collected over 24 hours to determine end products of catecholamine metabolism (epinephrine and norepinephrine)
   b. Nursing interventions/responsibilities: note medications, previous tests, and medical conditions that might interfere with test; restrict foods that contain vanilla, coffee, tea, citrus fruits, bananas, nuts, and chocolate for 3 days before 24-hour urine collection
10. Basal metabolic rate (BMR)
   a. Definition/purpose: noninvasive, indirect measurement of oxygen consumed by the body during a given time
   b. Nursing interventions/responsibilities: note medications taken before procedure; note environmental and emotional stressors

11. Visual acuity and field testing
    a. Definition/purpose: measurement of central and peripheral vision
    b. Nursing interventions/responsibilities: request patient to wear or bring corrective lenses; before procedure, assess patient's hearing and ability to follow directions
12. Computerized tomography (CT)
    a. Definition/purpose: noninvasive scan that may use I.V. injection of contrast dye to visualize the sella turcica and abdomen
    b. Nursing interventions/responsibilities: before procedure, explain the procedure; assess allergies to iodine, seafood, and radiopaque dye; allay anxiety; inform patient he may feel flushing of the face and throat irritation
13. Ultrasonography
    a. Definition/purpose: noninvasive examination that uses echoes from sound waves to visualize thyroid, pelvis, and abdomen
    b. Nursing interventions/responsibilities: before procedure, withhold food and fluids 8 to 12 hours before test; assess patient's ability to lie still; ask patient not to smoke or chew gum; administer enema as ordered; remove abdominal dressing
14. Closed percutaneous thyroid biopsy
    a. Definition/purpose: percutaneous, sterile aspiration of small amount of thyroid tissue for histologic evaluation
    b. Nursing interventions/responsibilities: before procedure, withhold food and fluids after midnight; obtain written, informed consent; after procedure, maintain bed rest for 24 hours; monitor VS; assess biopsy site for bleeding; assess patient for esophageal or tracheal puncture
15. Thyroid uptake (Radioactive iodine uptake: RAIU)
    a. Definition/purpose: measurement of amount of radioactive iodine taken up by the thyroid gland 24 hours after oral or I.V. administration of radioactive iodine
    b. Nursing interventions/responsibilities: before procedure, advise patient not to eat iodine-rich foods; discontinue all thyroid and cough medications 7 to 10 days before test; schedule scan before tests using iodine-based dyes
16. Thyroid scan
    a. Definition/purpose: visual imaging of distribution of radioactivity in the thyroid gland after oral or I.V. administration of radioactive isotope
    b. Nursing interventions/responsibilities: before procedure, advise patient not to eat iodine-rich foods; discontinue all thyroid and cough medications 7 to 10 days before test; schedule scan before tests using iodine-based dyes or radioactive iodine
17. Arteriography
    a. Definition/purpose: fluoroscopic examination of the arterial blood supply to the parathyroid, adrenal, or pancreatic glands after injection of a radiopaque dye through a catheter

b. Nursing interventions/responsibilities: before procedure, obtain written, informed consent; assess allergies to radiopaque dyes, iodine, and seafood; instruct patient he may feel flushing of the face and throat irritation after the dye injection; withhold food and fluids after midnight; after procedure, monitor VS, assess insertion site for bleeding

18. Sulkowitch's test
   a. Definition/purpose: laboratory analysis of urine to measure amount of calcium being excreted
   b. Nursing interventions/responsibilities: if hypercalcemia is suspected, collect a single urine sample before a meal; if hypocalcemia is suspected, collect a single urine sample after a meal

D. Possible psychosocial impact of endocrine disorders
1. Developmental impact
   a. Decreased self-esteem
   b. Changes in body image
   c. Embarrassment from the change in body function and structure
2. Economic impact
   a. Disruption of employment
   b. Cost of vocational retraining
   c. Cost of medications
   d. Cost of special diet
   e. Cost of hospitalizations and follow-up care
3. Occupational and recreational impact
   a. Physical activity restrictions
   b. Adjustment to change in occupation
4. Social impact
   a. Social withdrawal and isolation
   b. Change in eating patterns
   c. Change in role performance
   d. Change in sexual function

E. Possible risk factors for development of endocrine disorders
1. Modifiable risk factors
   a. Medication
   b. Stress
   c. Diet
   d. Obesity
2. Nonmodifiable risk factors
   a. Family history of endocrine illness
   b. History of trauma
   c. Aging process

F. Possible nursing diagnoses for patients with endocrine disorders
1. Actual nursing diagnoses
   a. Alteration in fluid volume: excess
   b. Fluid volume deficit

      c. Alteration in nutrition: more than body requirements

      d. Disturbance in self-concept: body image

      e. Alteration in patterns of urinary elimination

  2. Potential nursing diagnoses

      a. Potential for injury

      b. Social isolation

      c. Knowledge deficit

      d. Noncompliance

      e. Sensory-perceptual alteration: visual

      f. Sensory-perceptual alteration: tactile

      g. Impairment of skin integrity

      h. Alteration in thought process

G. Surgical intervention: adrenalectomy

  1. Definition: surgical removal of one or both adrenal glands

  2. Preoperative surgical nursing interventions/responsibilities

      a. Complete patient and family preoperative teaching: assess understanding of surgical procedure; explain operating room (OR), recovery room (RR), preoperative and postoperative routine; demonstrate postoperative turning, coughing, and deep breathing (TCDB), splinting, leg exercises, and range-of-motion (ROM) exercises; explain postoperative need for drainage tubes, surgical dressings, oxygen therapy, I.V. therapy, and pain control

      b. Complete preoperative check list

      c. Administer preoperative medications

      d. Allay patient and family anxiety about surgery

      e. Document patient history and physical assessment data base

      f. Administer steroids

      g. Administer vasopressors

  3. Postoperative surgical nursing interventions/responsibilities

      a. Assess cardiac, respiratory, neurologic status, and fluid balance

      b. Assess pain and administer postoperative analgesic

      c. Progress diet as tolerated

      d. Administer I.V. fluids

      e. Allay anxiety

      f. Assess surgical dressing and change as directed

      g. Reinforce TCDB and splinting of incision

      h. Maintain semi-Fowler position

      i. Assess for return of peristalsis

      j. Provide pulmonary toilet: incentive spirometry

      k. Maintain activity as tolerated

      l. Monitor VS, urinary output (UO), intake and output (I/O), central venous pressure (CVP), laboratory studies, EKG, neurovital signs, daily weights, specific gravity, urine for glucose and ketones

      m. Monitor and maintain position and patency of drainage tubes: nasogastric (NG), Foley, wound drainage

      n. Encourage ventilation of feelings about change in body image, need for lifelong medication replacement

      o. Administer antacids

      p. Maintain a quiet environment

      q. Administer hormone replacements

      r. Administer vasopressors

4. Possible surgical complications

      a. Shock

      b. Hypoglycemia

      c. Hemorrhage

      d. Peptic ulcers

      e. Adrenal crisis

      f. Pneumothorax

      g. Acute renal failure

      h. Infection

5. Patient/family postoperative teaching goals; the patient will:

      a. Keep follow-up appointments

      b. Maintain ideal weight

      c. State the action, side effects, and scheduling of medications

      d. Recognize the signs and symptoms of infection, hypovolemia, and hypoglycemia

      e. Avoid exposure to people with infections

      f. Alternate rest periods with activity

      g. Complete daily incision care

      h. Comply with lifelong hormone replacement

      i. Identify and reduce stress

      j. Wear medical identification bracelet

      k. Monitor blood pressure daily

      l. Explore methods to reduce insomnia

      m. Avoid extreme temperatures

H. Surgical intervention: hypophysectomy

1. Definition: surgical removal of part or all of the pituitary gland

2. Preoperative surgical nursing interventions/responsibilities

      a. Complete patient and family preoperative teaching: assess understanding of surgical procedure; explain OR, RR, preoperative and postoperative routine; demonstrate postoperative TCDB, splinting, leg exercises, and ROM; explain postoperative need for drainage tubes, surgical dressings, oxygen therapy, I.V. therapy, and pain control

      b. Complete preoperative check list

      c. Administer preoperative medications

      d. Allay patient and family anxiety about surgery

      e. Document patient history and physical assessment data base

      f. Administer steroids

      g. Administer antibiotics

3. Postoperative surgical nursing interventions/responsibilities
    a. Assess cardiac, respiratory, neurologic status, and fluid balance
    b. Assess pain and administer postoperative analgesic
    c. Progress diet as tolerated
    d. Administer I.V. fluids
    e. Allay anxiety
    f. Assess surgical dressing or nasal drip pad and change as directed
    g. Reinforce TCDB
    h. Maintain semi-Fowler position
    i. Assess for return of peristalsis
    j. Provide pulmonary toilet: incentive spirometry
    k. Maintain activity: as tolerated
    l. Monitor VS, UO, I/O, CVP, laboratory studies, neurovital signs, daily weights, specific gravity, urine glucose and ketones
    m. Monitor and maintain position and patency of Foley catheter
    n. Precautions: seizure
    o. Encourage ventilation of feelings about change in body image, fear of dying
    p. Administer antibiotics
    q. Administer hormone replacements
    r. Assess for signs of increased intracranial pressure (ICP)
    s. Assess for rhinorrhea
    t. Provide mouth and eye care
    u. Avoid brushing teeth
    v. Administer stool softeners
4. Possible surgical complications
    a. Diabetes insipidus
    b. Increased ICP
    c. Hemorrhage
    d. Adrenal crisis
    e. Thyroid storm
    f. Meningitis
    g. Diplopia
5. Patient/family postoperative teaching goals; the patient will:
    a. Keep follow-up appointments
    b. State the action, side effects, and scheduling of medications
    c. Recognize the signs and symptoms of infection, seizure activity, and hormone deficiencies
    d. Avoid coughing, blowing nose, lifting, straining at stool, sneezing
    e. Wear medical identification bracelet
    f. Comply with lifelong hormone replacement

I. **Surgical intervention: parathyroid surgeries**
    1. Definition
        a. Thyroidectomy: surgical removal of part or all of the thyroid gland
        b. Parathyroidectomy: surgical removal of one or more parathyroid glands

2. Preoperative surgical nursing interventions/responsibilities
   a. Complete patient and family preoperative teaching: assess understanding of surgical procedure; explain OR, RR, preoperative and postoperative routine; demonstrate postoperative TCDB, splinting, leg exercises, and ROM; explain postoperative need for drainage tubes, surgical dressings, oxygen therapy, I.V. therapy, and pain control
   b. Complete preoperative check list
   c. Administer preoperative medications
   d. Allay patient and family anxiety about surgery
   e. Document patient history and physical assessment data base
   f. Administer iodine preparations and antithyroid medications
3. Postoperative surgical nursing interventions/responsibilities
   a. Assess respiratory status
   b. Assess pain and administer postoperative analgesic
   c. Progress diet as tolerated
   d. Administer I.V. fluids
   e. Allay anxiety
   f. Assess surgical dressing for bleeding, especially at back of neck, and change dressing as directed
   g. Reinforce TCDB and splinting of incision
   h. Maintain semi-Fowler position, with neutral alignment and support to neck
   i. Assess for return of peristalsis
   j. Provide pulmonary toilet: incentive spirometry
   k. Maintain activity as tolerated
   l. Provide humidified cold steam nebulizer
   m. Monitor VS, UO, I/O, CVP, laboratory studies, urine glucose and ketones
   n. Monitor and maintain position and patency of wound drainage tubes
   o. Precautions: seizure
   p. Encourage ventilation of feelings about fear of choking, loss of voice
   q. Assess for tetany
   r. Assess for hoarseness and aphasia
   s. Assess for thyroid storm
   t. Discourage talking
   u. Have calcium gluconate and tracheostomy tray available
   v. Parathyroidectomy: provide high-calcium diet with vitamin D, administer calcium and vitamin D supplements
4. Possible surgical complications
   a. Hypocalcemia
   b. Laryngeal nerve damage
   c. Hypothyroidism
   d. Respiratory distress
   e. Hemorrhage
   f. Dysrhythmias

5. Patient/family postoperative teaching goals; the patient will:
   a. Keep follow-up appointments
   b. State the action, side effects, and scheduling of medications
   c. Recognize the signs and symptoms of infection, seizure activity, and hypothyroidism
   d. Alternate periods of talking with voice rest
   e. Complete daily incision care
   f. Complete daily ROM to the neck

J. Hyperthyroidism
   1. Definition: increased synthesis of thyroid hormone from overactivity (Graves' disease) or change in thyroid gland (toxic nodular goiter)
   2. Possible etiology
      a. Autoimmune disease
      b. Genetic
      c. Psychological or physiologic stress
      d. Thyroid adenomas
      e. Pituitary tumors
      f. Infection
   3. Pathophysiology
      a. Thyroid-stimulating antibodies (TSAb) have slow, sustained, stimulating effect on thyroid metabolism
      b. Accelerated metabolism causes increased synthesis of thyroid hormone
   4. Possible clinical manifestations
      a. Anxiety
      b. Flushed, smoooth skin
      c. Heat intolerance
      d. Mood swings
      e. Diaphoresis
      f. Tachycardia
      g. Palpitations
      h. Dyspnea
      i. Weakness
      j. Increased hunger
      k. Increased systolic blood pressure
      l. Tachypnea
      m. Fine hand tremors
      n. Exophthalmos
      o. Weight loss
      p. Diarrhea
      q. Hyperhydrosis
      r. Bruit or thrill over thyroid
   5. Possible diagnostic test findings
      a. Thyroid scan: presence of nodules
      b. Blood chemistry: increased T3, T4, PBI, Iodine 131; decreased TSH, cholesterol

    c. Electrocardiogram (EKG): atrial fibrillation

    d. BMR: increased

6. Medical management

    a. Diet therapy: high-protein, high-carbohydrate, high-calorie, with restriction of stimulants

    b. I.V. therapy: heparin lock

    c. Activity: bed rest

    d. Monitoring: VS, I/O

    e. Laboratory studies: T3, T4

    f. Sedatives: phenobarbitol (Luminal)

    g. Radiation therapy

    h. Thionamides: metimazole (Tapazole), propylthiouracil (PTU)

    i. Iodine preparations: potassium iodide (SSKI), radioactive iodine (Lugol's solution)

    j. Adrenergic blocking agents: propranolol (Inderal), reserpine (Serpasil), guanethidine sulfate (Ismelin)

    k. Vitamins: thiamine (vitamin B_1), ascorbic acid (vitamin C)

    l. Cardiac glycosides: digitalis (Lanoxin)

    m. Tranquilizers: diazepam (Valium), chlordiazepoxide (Librium)

    n. Glucocorticoids: cortisone acetate (Cortone), hydrocortisone sodium succinate (Solu-Cortef)

    o. I.V. glucose

7. Medical nursing interventions/responsibilities

    a. Maintain diet

    b. Avoid stimulants

    c. Administer I.V. fluids

    d. Assess fluid balance

    e. Monitor and record VS, UO, I/O, laboratory studies

    f. Administer medications

    g. Weigh daily

    h. Provide rest periods

    i. Povide a quiet, cool environment

    j. Administer eye and skin care

    k. Allay anxiety

    l. Encourage ventilation of feelings about change in body image

    m. Provide postchemotherapeutic and/or postradiation nursing care: provide skin, mouth, and perineal care; encourage dietary intake; administer antiemetics and antidiarrheals; monitor for bleeding, infection, and electrolyte imbalance; provide rest periods

8. Patient/family teaching goals; the patient will:

    a. Keep follow-up appointments

    b. Stop smoking

    c. Maintain ideal weight

    d. State the action, side effects, and scheduling of medications

    e. Identify and reduce stress

f. Recognize the signs and symptoms of thyroid storm
g. Adhere to activity limitations
h. Avoid exposure to people with infections
i. Alternate rest periods with activity
j. Monitor self for infection
k. Follow dietary recommendations and restrictions
l. Maintain a quiet environment
m. State reasons for emotional lability

9. Possible medical complications
    a. Thyroid storm (thyroid crisis): tachycardia, delirium, agitation, coma, death, hyperpyrexia, dehydration, dysrhythmias, diarrhea
    b. Cardiac dysrhythmias
    c. Diabetes mellitus

10. Possible surgical interventions: subtotal thyroidectomy when euthyroid state established (see page 163)

K. **Hypothyroidism (myxedema)**
1. Definition: underactive state of thyroid gland, resulting in absence or decreased secretion of thyroid hormone
2. Possible etiology
    a. Autoimmune disease: Hashimoto's thyroiditis
    b. Thyroidectomy
    c. Overuse of antithyroid drugs
    d. Malfunction of pituitary gland
    e. Use of radioactive iodine
3. Pathophysiology
    a. Thyroid gland fails to secrete satisfactory quantity of thyroid hormone
    b. Hyposecretion of thyroid hormone results in overall decrease in metabolism
4. Possible clinical manifestations
    a. Fatigue
    b. Weight gain
    c. Dry, flaky skin
    d. Edema
    e. Cold intolerance
    f. Coarse hair
    g. Alopecia
    h. Thick tongue, swollen lips
    i. Mental sluggishness
    j. Menstrual disorders
    k. Constipation
    l. Hypersensitivity to narcotics, barbiturates, and anesthetics
    m. Anorexia
    n. Decreased diaphoresis
    o. Hypothermia

5. Possible diagnostic test findings
   a. Blood chemistry: decreased T3, T4, PBI, sodium; increased TSH, cholesterol
   b. BMR: decreased
   c. RAIU: decreased
   d. EKG: sinus bradycardia
6. Medical management
   a. Diet therapy: high-fiber, high-protein, low-calorie, with increased fluid intake
   b. Activity: as tolerated
   c. Monitoring: VS, UO, I/O
   d. Laboratory studies: T3, T4, sodium
   e. Stool softeners: docusate sodium (Colace)
   f. Thyroid hormone replacement: levothyroxine (Synthroid), liothyronine sodium (Cytomel), thyroglobulin (Proloid)
7. Medical nursing interventions/responsibilities
   a. Maintain diet
   b. Force fluids
   c. Assess fluid balance
   d. Monitor and record VS, UO, I/O, laboratory studies
   e. Administer medications
   f. Encourage ventilation of feelings of depression
   g. Encourage physical activity and mental stimulation
   h. Provide a warm environment
   i. Avoid sedation: administer one-half to one-third the normal dose of sedatives or narcotics
   j. Assess for constipation, infection, and edema
   k. Prevent skin breakdown
   l. Provide frequent rest periods
8. Patient/family teaching goals; the patient will:
   a. Keep follow-up appointments
   b. Maintain regular exercise program
   c. Maintain ideal weight
   d. State the action, side effects, and scheduling of medications
   e. Recognize the signs and symptoms of myxedema coma
   f. Alternate rest periods with activity
   g. Monitor self for constipation
   h. Follow dietary recommendations and restrictions
   i. Use additional protection and limit activity in cold weather
   j. Avoid use of sedatives
   k. Complete daily skin care
9. Possible medical complications
   a. Coronary artery disease
   b. Congestive heart failure (CHF)
   c. Acute organic psychosis
   d. Angina

e. Myocardial infarction (MI)

f. Myxedema coma: hypoventilation, hypothermia, respiratory acidosis, syncope, bradycardia, hypotension, convulsions, and cerebral hypoxia

10. Possible surgical interventions: none

L. Thyroid cancer

1. Definition: malignant, primary tumor of the thyroid, which does not affect thyroid hormone secretion

2. Possible etiology
   a. Chronic overstimulation of the pituitary gland
   b. Chronic overstimulation of the thymus gland
   c. Neck radiation

3. Pathophysiology
   a. Unregulated cell growth and uncontrolled cell division result in the development of a neoplasm
   b. Papillary carcinoma: well-differentiated columnar cells form a solitary nodule in the thyroid gland that spreads to the cervical lymph nodes
   c. Follicular carcinoma: encapsulated, well-differentiated cells that invade blood vessels and lymphatics
   d. Anaplastic carcinoma: either squamous, spindle, or small round cells
   e. Medullary carcinoma: solid, differentiated tumor arising from calcitonin-producing C-cells

4. Possible clinical manifestations
   a. Enlarged thyroid gland
   b. Painless, firm, irregular, and enlarged thyroid nodule or mass
   c. Palpable cervical lymph nodes
   d. Dysphagia
   e. Hoarseness
   f. Dyspnea

5. Possible diagnostic test findings
   a. RAIU: presence of "cold" nodule
   b. Thyroid biopsy: cytology positive for cancer cells
   c. Thyroid function tests: normal
   d. Blood chemistry: increased calcitonin, serotonin, and prostaglandins

6. Medical management
   a. Diet therapy: high-protein, high-carbohydrate, high-calorie, with supplemental feedings
   b. I.V. therapy: heparin lock
   c. Activity: as tolerated
   d. Monitoring: VS, I/O
   e. Laboratory studies: calcitonin, serotonin
   f. Radiation therapy
   g. Chemotherapy: chlorambucil (Leukeran), doxorubicin hydrochloride (Adriamycin), vincristine sulfate (Oncovin)
   h. Thyroid hormone replacement: levothyroxine (Synthroid), liothyronine sodium (Cytomel), thyroglobulin (Proloid)

7. Medical nursing interventions/responsibilities
   a. Maintain diet
   b. Assess respiratory status
   c. Assess ability to swallow
   d. Monitor and record VS, I/O, laboratory studies
   e. Administer medications
   f. Encourage ventilation of feelings about fear of dying
   g. Provide postchemotherapeutic and/or postradiation nursing care: provide skin, mouth, and perineal care; encourage dietary intake; administer antiemetics and antidiarrheals; monitor for bleeding, infection, and electrolyte imbalance; provide rest periods
8. Patient/family teaching goals; the patient will:
   a. Keep follow-up appointments
   b. Maintain ideal weight
   c. State the action, side effects, and scheduling of medications
   d. Recognize the signs and symptoms of respiratory distress and difficulty swallowing
   e. Alternate rest periods with activity
   f. Follow dietary recommendations and restrictions
   g. Seek help from community agencies and resources
9. Possible medical complications
   a. Laryngotracheal obstruction
   b. Respiratory distress
   c. Esophageal obstruction
10. Possible surgical interventions
   a. Thyroidectomy (see page 163)
   b. Modified neck dissection

M. Simple goiter
1. Definition: enlarged thyroid gland
2. Possible etiology
   a. Decreased iodine intake
   b. Intake of goitrogenic foods: soybeans, peanuts, peaches, strawberries
   c. Use of goitrogenic drugs: iodine, lithium, propylthiouracil
   d. Genetic defects
3. Pathophysiology
   a. Low levels of thyroid hormone stimulate increased secretion of TSH by the pituitary gland
   b. TSH stimulation causes the thyroid to increase in size to compensate for the low levels of thyroid hormone
4. Possible clinical manifestations
   a. Dysphagia
   b. Enlarged thyroid gland
   c. Dyspnea

5. Possible diagnostic test findings
   a. Blood chemistry: normal or decreased T4
   b. RAIU: normal or increased
6. Medical management
   a. Diet therapy: avoid goitrogenic foods, use iodized salt
   b. Activity: as tolerated
   c. Monitoring: VS, I/O
   d. Laboratory studies: T4
   e. Iodine preparations: potassium iodide (SSKI), radioactive iodine (Lugol's solution)
   f. Thyroid hormone replacement: levothyroxine (Synthroid), liothyronine sodium (Cytomel), thyroglobulin (Proloid)
   g. Avoid goitrogenic drugs
7. Medical nursing interventions/responsibilities
   a. Maintain diet
   b. Assess respiratory status
   c. Monitor and record VS, I/O, laboratory studies
   d. Administer medications
   e. Encourage ventilation of feelings about change in body image
   f. Assess ability to swallow
8. Patient/family teaching goals; the patient will:
   a. Keep follow-up appointments
   b. State the action, side effects, and scheduling of medications
   c. Recognize the signs and symptoms of respiratory distress and difficulty swallowing
   d. Follow dietary recommendations and restrictions
9. Possible medical complications
   a. Respiratory distress
   b. Laryngotracheal obstruction
10. Possible surgical interventions: subtotal thyroidectomy (see page 163)

N. **Hyperparathyroidism**
   1. Definition: overactivity of one or more parathyroid glands, resulting in increased PTH secretion
   2. Possible etiology
      a. Chronic renal failure
      b. Bone disease
      c. Benign adenomas
      d. Hypertrophy of parathyroid gland
      e. Malignant tumors of parathyroid gland
      f. Vitamin D deficiency
      g. Malabsorption
   3. Pathophysiology
      a. Excessive secretion of PTH leads to bone demineralization and hypocalcemia
      b. Hypercalcemia increases the risk of renal calculi

4. Possible clinical manifestations
   a. Renal colic
   b. Renal calculi
   c. Dysrhythmias
   d. Constipation
   e. Bowel obstruction
   f. Anorexia
   g. Weight loss
   h. Nausea and vomiting
   i. Depression
   j. Mental dullness
   k. Fatigue
   l. Osteoporosis
   m. Muscle weakness
   n. Mood swings
   o. Deep bone pain
   p. Hematuria
   q. Paresthesia
   r. Thick nails
   s. Pathologic fractures
5. Possible diagnostic test findings
   a. EKG: shortened QT interval
   b. Urine chemistry: decreased phosphorus; increased calcium
   c. Blood chemistry: increased calcium, BUN, creatinine, chloride, alkaline phosphatase; decreased phosphorus
   d. X-ray: osteoporosis
6. Medical management
   a. Diet therapy: low-calcium, high-fiber, high-phosphorus, in small frequent feedings, with increased fluid intake to 3,000 ml/day
   b. I.V. therapy: heparin lock
   c. Activity: ad lib
   d. Monitoring: VS, UO, I/O
   e. Laboratory studies: calcium, phosphorus, BUN, creatinine, potassium, sodium
   f. Radiation therapy
   g. Treatments: strain urine, bed cradle
   h. Analgesics: oxycodone hydrochloride (Tylox)
   i. Diuretics: furosemide (Lasix), ethacrynic acid (Edecrin)
   j. Antacids: aluminum hydroxide gel (Alternagel)
   k. Estrogens: estrogen (Premarin)
   l. Antineoplastics: plicamycin (Mithracin)
   m. Phosphate salts: K-Phos, Neutra-Phos
   n. Dialysis using calcium-free dialysate
   o. I.V. saline

7. Medical nursing interventions/responsibilities
   a. Maintain diet
   b. Force fluids with acidifying solutions: cranberry juice
   c. Administer I.V. fluids
   d. Assess urinary status
   e. Monitor and record VS, UO, I/O, laboratory studies
   f. Administer medications
   g. Encourage ventilation of feelings about chronic illness
   h. Encourage ambulation
   i. Prevent falls
   j. Strain urine
   k. Assess bone, flank pain
   l. Move patient carefully to prevent pathologic fractures
   m. Limit strenuous activity
   n. Assess for constipation
   o. Provide postchemotherapeutic and/or postradiation nursing care: provide skin, mouth, and perineal care; encourage dietary intake; administer antiemetics and antidiarrheals; monitor for bleeding, infection, and electrolyte imbalance; provide rest periods
8. Patient/family teaching goals; the patient will:
   a. Keep follow-up appointments
   b. Maintain regular exercise program
   c. Maintain ideal weight
   d. State the action, side effects, and scheduling of medications
   e. Recognize the signs and symptoms of renal calculi
   f. Adhere to activity limitations
   g. Alternate rest periods with activity
   h. Follow dietary recommendations and restrictions
   i. Promote a safe environment
   j. Strain urine
   k. Prevent falls
   l. Prevent constipation
9. Possible medical complications
   a. Peptic ulcer
   b. Psychosis
   c. Dysrhythmias
   d. Renal failure
   e. Pathologic fractures
10. Possible surgical interventions: parathyroidectomy (see page 163)

O. Hypoparathyroidism
1. Definition: decrease in PTH secretion
2. Possible etiology
   a. Thyroidectomy
   b. Autoimmune disease

   c. Parathyroidectomy
   d. Radiation
   e. Use of radioactive iodine
   f. Parathyroid tumor
3. Pathophysiology
   a. Decreased PTH decreases stimulation to osteoclasts, resulting in decreased release of calcium and phosphorus from bone
   b. Gastrointestinal absorption of calcium is decreased while absorption of phosphorus is increased with decreased circulating PTH
   c. Decreased blood calcium causes a rise in serum phosphates and decreased phosphate excretion by the kidney
4. Possible clinical manifestations
   a. Lethargy
   b. Calcification of ocular lens
   c. Muscle and abdominal spasms
   d. Trousseau's sign: positive
   e. Chvostek's sign: positive
   f. Tingling of fingers
   g. Dysrhythmias
   h. Convulsions
   i. Visual disturbances: diplopia, photophobia, blurring
   j. Dyspnea
   k. Laryngeal stridor
   l. Personality changes
   m. Brittle nails
   n. Alopecia
   o. Deep tendon reflexes: increased
5. Possible diagnostic test findings
   a. Blood chemistry: decreased PTH, calcium; increased phosphorus
   b. Urine chemistry: decreased calcium
   c. X-ray: calcification of basal ganglia; increased bone density
   d. EKG: prolonged QT interval
   e. Sulkowitch's test: decreased
6. Medical management
   a. Diet therapy: high-calcium, low-phosphorus, low-sodium, with spinach restriction
   b. Activity: as tolerated
   c. I.V. therapy: heparin lock
   d. Monitoring: VS, UO, I/O
   e. Laboratory studies: PTH, calcium, phosphorus
   f. Precautions: seizure
   g. Antacids: aluminum hydroxide gel (Alternagel)
   h. Sedatives: phenobarbital (Luminal)
   i. Anticonvulsants: phenytoin sodium (Dilantin), $MgSO_4$ (Epsom salt)
   j. Vitamins: ergocalciferol (vitamin D), dihydrotachysterol (Hytakerol)

    k. Oral calcium salts: calcium gluconate (Kalcinate), calcium carbonate (Os-Cal)

    l. Diuretic: chlorthalidone (Hygroton)

    m. Hormone replacement: parathyroid extract (parathormone)

    n. I.V. calcium salts: calcium chloride or calcium gluconate

7. Medical nursing interventions/responsibilities

    a. Maintain diet

    b. Assess neurologic status

    c. Maintain seizure precautions

    d. Monitor and record VS, I/O, laboratory studies

    e. Administer medications

    f. Allay anxiety

    g. Keep tracheostomy tray and I.V. calcium gluconate available

    h. Maintain a calm environment

8. Patient/family teaching goals; the patient will:

    a. Keep follow-up appointments

    b. State the action, side effects, and scheduling of medications

    c. Identify and reduce stress

    d. Recognize the signs and symptoms of seizure activity

    e. Follow dietary recommendations and restrictions

    f. Promote a safe environment

    g. Maintain a quiet environment

9. Possible medical complications

    a. CHF

    b. Mental retardation

    c. Blindness

10. Possible surgical interventions: none

P. Cushing's syndrome (hypercortisolism)

1. Definition

    a. Hyperactivity of the adrenal cortex that results in excessive secretion of glucocorticoid, particularly cortisol

    b. Possible increase in mineralocorticoids and sex hormones

2. Possible etiology

    a. Hyperplasia of adrenal glands

    b. Hypothalamic stimulation of pituitary gland

    c. Adenoma or carcinoma of pituitary gland

    d. Exogenous secretion of ACTH by malignant neoplasms in lung or gall bladder

    e. Excessive or prolonged administration of glucocorticoids or ACTH

    f. Adenoma or carcinoma of adrenal cortex

3. Pathophysiology

    a. Hypothalamic stimulation of pituitary gland causes excessive secretion of ACTH

    b. Excessive secretion of ACTH causes increased plasma cortisol

    c. Secretion of hypothalamic corticotropin-regulatory hormone (CRH) is not diminished by elevated blood cortisol levels

4. Possible clinical manifestations
   a. Weight gain
   b. Hirsutism
   c. Amenorrhea
   d. Weakness and fatigue
   e. Pain in joints
   f. Ecchymosis
   g. Edema
   h. Hypertension
   i. Mood swings
   j. Fragile skin
   k. Purple striae on abdomen
   l. Poor wound healing
   m. Truncal obesity
   n. Buffalo hump
   o. Moon face
   p. Gynecomastia
   q. Enlarged clitoris
   r. Decreased libido
   s. Muscle wasting
   t. Recurrent infections
   u. Acne

5. Possible diagnostic test findings
   a. Dexamethasone suppression test: no decrease in 17-OHCS
   b. X-ray: presence of pituitary or adrenal tumor; osteoporosis
   c. Angiography: presence of pituitary or adrenal tumors
   d. CT scan: presence of pituitary or adrenal tumors
   e. Urine chemistry: increased 17-OCHS and 17-KS; decreased specific gravity; glycosuria
   f. Blood chemistry: increased cortisol, aldosterone, sodium, ACTH; decreased potassium
   g. Ultrasonography: presence of pituitary or adrenal tumors
   h. Hematology: increased WBC, RBC; decreased eosinophils
   i. GTT: hyperglycemia

6. Medical management
   a. Diet therapy: low-sodium, low-carbohydrate, low-calorie, high-potassium, high-protein
   b. Activity: as tolerated
   c. Monitoring: VS, I/O, UO, urine glucose and ketones, specific gravity
   d. Laboratory studies: sodium, potassium, cortisol, BUN, glucose, WBC, RBC
   e. Radiation therapy
   f. Chemotherapy
   g. Diuretics: furosemide (Lasix), ethacrynic acid (Edecrin)

      h. Potassium supplements: potassium chloride (K-Lor), potassium gluconate (Kaon)

      i. Adrenal suppressants: metyrapone (Metopirone), aminoglutethamide (Cytadren)

      j. Antineoplastics: mitotane (Lysodren)

7. Medical nursing interventions/responsibilities

      a. Maintain diet

      b. Assess fluid balance

      c. Monitor and record VS, UO, I/O, specific gravity, finger sticks, urine glucose and ketones, laboratory studies

      d. Assess edema

      e. Assess for infections of skin, respiratory, and urinary tracts

      f. Protect from falls and bruising

      g. Protect from infection

      h. Provide meticulous skin care

      i. Limit water intake

      j. Weigh daily

      k. Administer medications

      l. Encourage ventilation of feelings about change in body image and sexual function

      m. Provide rest periods

      n. Minimize environmental stress

      o. Provide postchemotherapeutic and/or postradiation nursing care: provide skin, mouth, and perineal care; encourage dietary intake; administer antiemetics and antidiarrheals; monitor for bleeding, infection, and electrolyte imbalance; provide rest periods

8. Patient/family teaching goals; the patient will:

      a. Keep follow-up appointments

      b. Maintain ideal weight

      c. State the action, side effects, and scheduling of medications

      d. Identify and reduce stress

      e. Recognize the signs and symptoms of infection and fluid retention

      f. Adhere to activity limitations

      g. Avoid exposure to people with infections

      h. Alternate rest periods with activity

      i. Monitor self for infection

      j. Follow dietary recommendations and restrictions

      k. Promote a safe environment

      l. Maintain a quiet environment

      m. Wear medical identification bracelet

9. Possible medical complications

      a. Adrenal insufficiency

      b. Infection

      c. Peptic ulcers

      d. Hypertension

      e. Fractures

    f. CHF
    g. Psychosis
    h. Dysrhythmias
    i. Diabetes mellitus
    j. Arteriosclerosis
    k. Nephrosclerosis
10. Possible surgical interventions
    a. Adrenalectomy (see page 161)
    b. Hypophysectomy (see page 162)

Q. Addison's disease
1. Definition: chronic hypoactivity of the adrenal cortex, resulting in insufficient secretion of glucocorticoids (cortisol) and mineralocorticoids (aldosterone)
2. Possible etiology
    a. Idiopathic atrophy of adrenal glands
    b. Surgical removal of adrenal glands
    c. Autoimmune disease
    d. Tuberculosis
    e. Metastatic lesions from lung cancer
    f. Pituitary hypofunction
    g. Histoplasmosis
    h. Trauma
3. Pathophysiology
    a. Autoimmune theory: body produces adrenocorticol antibodies, resulting in adrenal hypofunction
    b. Decreased aldosterone causes disturbances in sodium, water, and potassium metabolism
    c. Decreased cortisol causes abnormal metabolism of fat, protein, and carbohydrate
4. Possible clinical manifestations
    a. Hypoglycemia
    b. Weakness and lethargy
    c. Bronzed skin pigmentation of nipples, scars, and buccal mucosa
    d. Dehydration
    e. Anorexia
    f. Thirst
    g. Decreased pubic and axillary hair
    h. Orthostatic hypotension
    i. Diarrhea
    j. Nausea
    k. Weight loss
    l. Depression
5. Possible diagnostic test findings
    a. Blood chemistry: decreased Hct, Hgb, cortisol, glucose, sodium, chloride aldosterone; increased BUN, potassium

b. Urine chemistry: decreased 17-KS and 17-OHCS
c. BMR: decreased
d. Fasting blood sugar (FBS): hypoglycemia
e. EKG: prolonged PR and QT intervals

6. Medical management
   a. Diet therapy: high-carbohydrate, high-protein, high-sodium, low-potassium, in small, frequent feedings before steroid therapy; high-potassium and low-sodium when on steroid therapy
   b. I.V. therapy: hydration, electrolyte replacement; heparin lock
   c. Activity: bed rest
   d. Monitoring: VS, UO, I/O, specific gravity
   e. Laboratory studies: sodium, potassium, osmolality, cortisol, chloride, glucose, BUN, Cr, Hgb, Hct
   f. I.V. saline
   g. Vasopressor: phenylephrine hydrochloride (NeoSynephrine)
   h. Antacids: Magnesium and aluminum hydroxide (Maalox), aluminum hydroxide gel (Gelusil)
   i. Mineralocorticoids (aldosterone): fludrocortisone acetate (Florinef)
   j. Glucocorticoids: cortisone acetate (Cortone), hydrocortisone (Solu-Cortef)

7. Medical nursing interventions/responsibilities
   a. Maintain diet
   b. Adminster I.V. fluids
   c. Assess fluid balance
   d. Monitor and record VS, UO, I/O, specific gravity, laboratory studies
   e. Weigh daily
   f. Administer medications
   g. Maintain bed rest
   h. Allay anxiety
   i. Assess edema
   j. Protect from falls
   k. Encourage fluid intake
   l. Assist with activities of daily living (ADL)
   m. Maintain a quiet environment
   n. Protect patient from infection

8. Patient/family teaching goals; the patient will:
   a. Keep follow-up appointments
   b. Avoid strenuous exercise, particularly in hot weather
   c. Maintain ideal weight
   d. State the action, side effects, and scheduling of medications
   e. Identify and reduce stress
   f. Recognize the signs and symptoms of adrenal crisis
   g. Avoid exposure to people with infections
   h. Alternate rest periods with activity
   i. Monitor self for infection

j. Follow dietary recommendations and restrictions
k. Maintain a quiet environment
l. Increase fluid intake in hot weather
m. Avoid use of over-the-counter drugs
n. Wear medical identification bracelet
9. Possible medical complications
   a. Addisonian crisis (adrenal crisis): marked hypotension, cyanosis, abdominal cramps, diarrhea, costovertebral tenderness, fever, confusion, coma
   b. Dysrhythmias
   c. Hypovolemic shock
   d. Renal failure
10. Possible surgical interventions: none

R. Pheochromocytoma
1. Definition: catecholamine-secreting neoplasm associated with hyperfunctioning adrenal medulla
2. Possible etiology
   a. Genetics
   b. Pregnancy
   c. Trauma
3. Pathophysiology
   a. Tumor in the adrenal medulla secretes large amounts of catecholamines (epinephrine and norepinephrine)
   b. Increased catecholamines cause hypertension, increased BMR, and hyperglycemia
4. Possible clinical manifestations
   a. Labile malignant hypertension
   b. Throbbing headaches
   c. Diaphoresis
   d. Palpitations
   e. Tachycardia
   f. Excessive anxiety
   g. Hyperactivity
   h. Dilated pupils
   i. Cold extremities
   j. Weakness
   k. Weight loss
   l. Dyspnea
   m. Vertigo
   n. Angina
   o. Nausea
   p. Vomiting
   q. Anorexia
   r. Visual disturbances
   s. Polyuria

      t. Diarrhea
      u. Tinnitus
      v. Tremors

5. Possible diagnostic test findings
      a. CT scan: presence of adrenal tumor
      b. Angiography: presence of adrenal tumor
      c. BMR: increased
      d. VMA: increased
      e. EKG: tachycardia
      f. Blood chemistries: increased BUN, Cr, glucose, catecholamines
      g. Urine chemistries: increased glucose and catecholamines

6. Medical management
      a. Diet therapy: high-calorie, high-vitamin and mineral, with restricted use of stimulants
      b. Activity: as tolerated
      c. Monitoring: VS, UO, I/O, urine glucose and ketones
      d. Position: semi-Fowler
      e. Laboratory studies: BUN, Cr, glucose
      f. Radiation therapy
      g. Sedatives: phenobarbital (Luminal)
      h. Alpha adrenergic blockers: phentolamine (Regitine), phenoxybenzamine hydrochloride (Dibenzyline)
      i. Beta adrenergic blockers: propranolol (Inderal)
      j. Vasodilators: nitroprusside sodium (Nipride)
      k. Tranquilizers: diazepam (Valium), chlordiazepoxide (Librium)
      l. Catecholamine inhibitors: metyrosine (Demser)

7. Medical nursing interventions/responsibilities
      a. Maintain diet
      b. Assess cardiovascular status
      c. Maintain semi-Fowler position
      d. Monitor and record VS, UO, I/O, orthostatic blood pressure, specific gravity, urine glucose and ketones, neurovital signs, laboratory studies
      e. Weigh daily
      f. Administer medications
      g. Encourage ventilation of feelings about fear of dying
      h. Protect from falls
      i. Minimize environmental stress
      j. Provide rest periods
      k. Keep phentolamine (Regitine) available

8. Patient/family teaching goals; the patient will:
      a. Keep follow-up appointments
      b. Stop smoking
      c. Maintain ideal weight
      d. State the action, side effects, and scheduling of medications
      e. Identify and reduce stress
      f. Recognize the signs and symptoms of renal failure

   g. Avoid exposure to people with infections
   h. Alternate rest periods with activity
   i. Monitor self for infection
   j. Follow dietary recommendations and restrictions
   k. Promote a safe environment
   l. Maintain a quiet environment
   m. Monitor blood pressure, urine glucose, and ketones daily
9. Possible medical complications
   a. Cardiac arrest
   b. Cerebral hemorrhage
   c. Blindness
   d. Renal failure
   e. MI
   f. CHF
10. Possible surgical interventions
    a. Adrenal medulla resection after administration of phentolamine (Regitine)
    b. Adrenalectomy (see page 161)

S. Hyperaldosteronism (primary aldosteronism, Conn's syndrome)

1. Definition: hypersecretion of aldosterone (mineralocorticoid) from adrenal cortex
2. Possible etiology
   a. Adenoma of adrenal cortex
   b. Adrenal hyperplasia
   c. Adrenal carcinoma
3. Pathophysiology: Aldosterone's primary effect on renal tubules causes kidneys to retain sodium and water and excrete potassium and hydrogen
4. Possible clinical manifestations
   a. Muscle weakness
   b. Polyuria
   c. Polydipsia
   d. Metabolic alkalosis
   e. Hypertension
   f. Postural hypotension
   g. Headache
   h. Paresthesia
   i. Pyelonephritis
   j. Nocturia
   k. Chvostek's sign: positive
   l. Trousseau's sign: positive
5. Possible diagnostic test findings
   a. Blood chemistry: decreased potassium; increased sodium, carbon dioxide (CO_2)
   b. Arterial blood gases (ABGs): metabolic alkalosis
   c. Urine chemistry: increased aldosterone, protein, pH; decreased specific gravity

6. Medical management
   a. Diet therapy: high-potassium, low-sodium
   b. Activity: as tolerated
   c. Monitoring: VS, U/O, I/O
   d. Laboratory studies: potassium, sodium, calcium, ABGs
   e. Potassium salts: potassium chloride (KCl), potassium gluconate (Kaon)
   f. Diuretics: spironolactone (Aldactone), acetazolamide (Diamox)
   g. Calcium salts: calcium gluconate (Kalcinate), calcium carbonate (Os-Cal)
7. Medical nursing interventions/responsibilities
   a. Maintain diet as tolerated
   b. Assess fluid balance
   c. Monitor and record VS, UO, I/O, orthostatic blood pressure, specific gravity laboratory studies
   d. Monitor laboratory results: ABGs, sodium, potassium, calcium
   e. Administer medications
   f. Allay anxiety
   g. Weigh daily
   h. Provide a quiet environment
8. Patient/family teaching goals; the patient will:
   a. Keep follow-up appointments
   b. Maintain ideal weight
   c. State the action, side effects, and scheduling of medications
   d. Recognize the signs and symptoms of fluid overload and muscle irritability
   e. Alternate rest periods with activity
   f. Follow dietary recommendations and restrictions
   g. Maintain a quiet environment
9. Possible medical complications
   a. Neuropathy
   b. Dysrhythmias
10. Possible surgical interventions: adrenalectomy (see page 161)

T. Diabetes mellitus
1. Definition
   a. Chronic disorder of carbohydrate metabolism with subsequent alteration of protein and fat metabolism
   b. Results from a disturbance in the production, action, and rate of utilization of insulin
   c. Type I (IDDM): insulin-dependent or ketosis-prone diabetes
   d. Type II (NIDDM): insulin-independent or ketosis-resistant diabetes
2. Possible etiology
   a. Failure of body to produce insulin
   b. Blockage of insulin supply
   c. Autoimmune disease
   d. Receptor defect in normally insulin-responsive cells

      e. Genetics
      f. Exposure to chemicals
      g. Hyperpituitarism
      h. Cushing's syndrome
      i. Hyperthyroidism
      j. Infection
      k. Surgery
      l. Stress

3. Pathophysiology
      a. Type I (IDDM) results from an inability to produce endogenous insulin by the beta cells in the islets of Langerhans in the pancreas
      b. Type II (NIDDM) is a deficit in insulin release or insulin-receptor defect in peripheral tissues
      c. Insulin deprivation of insulin-dependent cells leads to a marked decrease in the cellular rate of glucose uptake
      d. Glucogenesis increases because of decreased stimulation of glucose metabolism with resulting hyperglycemia and glycosuria
      e. Decreased insulin triggers release of free fatty acids that cannot be metabolized and are released as ketone bodies in blood urine
      f. Decreased insulin depresses protein synthesis, causing a release of amino acids that are converted by the liver into glucose and ketones
      g. The formation of urea results in overall nitrogen loss

4. Possible clinical manifestations
      a. Weight loss
      b. Anorexia
      c. Polyphagia
      d. Acetone breath
      e. Weakness
      f. Fatigue
      g. Dehydration
      h. Pain
      i. Paresthesia
      j. Polyuria
      k. Polydipsia
      l. Kussmaul respirations
      m. Multiple infections and boils
      n. Flushed, warm, smooth, shiny skin
      o. Atrophic muscles
      p. Poor wound healing
      q. Mottled extremities
      r. Peripheral and visceral neuropathies
      s. Retinopathy
      t. Sexual dysfunction
      u. Blurred vision

5. Possible diagnostic test findings
   a. Blood chemistry: increased glucose, potassium, chloride, ketones, cholesterol, triglycerides; decreased CO_2; pH less than 7.4
   b. Urine chemistry: increased glucose, ketones
   c. FBS: increased
   d. GTT: hyperglycemia
   e. Postprandial blood sugar: hyperglycemia
6. Medical management
   a. Diet therapy: individually prescribed diet based on ideal weight, metabolic activity, and personal activity levels; individual's caloric needs are designed to distribute carbohydrate, fat, and protein intake (ratio 2:1:1) over 24 hours using American Diabetes Association's exchange method; avoid refined and simple sugars and saturated fats; limit cholesterol
   b. Activity: as tolerated
   c. Monitoring: VS, UO, I/O
   d. Laboratory studies: glucose, potassium, pH
   e. Hypoglycemics: short-acting (regular, Semilente); intermediate-acting (NPH, Lente); long-acting (PZI, Ultralente); tolbutamide (Orinase), chlorpropamide (Diabinese), acetohexamide (Dymelor), tolazamide (Tolinase)
   f. Vitamin and mineral supplements
7. Medical nursing interventions/responsibilities
   a. Maintain diet
   b. Force fluids
   c. Assess acid-base and fluid balance
   d. Monitor and record VS, UO, I/O, urine glucose and ketones, finger sticks, laboratory studies
   e. Administer medications
   f. Encourage ventilation of feelings about diet and medication regime
   g. Encourage activity as tolerated
   h. Weigh weekly
   i. Provide meticulous skin and foot care
   j. Monitor patient for infection
   k. Maintain a warm and quiet environment
   l. Monitor wound healing
   m. Observe for Somogyi phenomena
8. Patient/family teaching goals; the patient will:
   a. Keep follow-up appointments
   b. Maintain regular exercise program
   c. Stop smoking
   d. Maintain ideal weight
   e. State the action, side effects, and scheduling of medications
   f. Identify and reduce stress
   g. Recognize the signs and symptoms of hyperglycemia and hypoglycemia

     h. Alternate rest periods with activity
     i. Monitor self for infection and skin breakdown
     j. Follow dietary recommendations and restrictions
     k. Maintain a quiet environment
     l. Seek help from community agencies and resources
     m. State proper dietary substitutions if unable to take prescribed diet because of illness
     n. Adjust diet and insulin for changes in work, exercise, trauma, infection, fever, and stress
     o. Demonstrate administration of hypoglycemics
     p. Demonstrate Clinitest, Acetest, and finger sticks
     q. Complete daily skin and foot care
     r. Wear medical identification bracelet
     s. Carry emergency supply of glucose
     t. Seek counseling for sexual dysfunction
     u. Avoid use of over-the-counter medication
     v. Avoid alcohol
9. Possible medical complications
     a. Ketoacidosis (diabetic coma): abdominal pain, acetone breath, altered consciousness, hot, flushed skin, Kussmaul respirations, nausea, vomiting, hypotension, oliguria, tachycardia
     b. Insulin reaction (hypoglycemia): hunger, weakness, hand tremors, pallor, tachycardia, diaphoresis, irritability, confusion, diplopia, slurred speech, headaches
     c. Infections
     d. Peripheral neuropathies
     e. Glaucoma
     f. Impotence
     g. Coronary artery disease
     h. Gangrene
     i. Cerebrovascular accident (CVA)
     j. Chronic renal failure
     k. Nonketotic hyperosmolar coma: severe dehydration, severe hypotension, fever, stupor, and seizures
10. Possible surgical interventions: none

U. Diabetes insipidus
1. Definition: deficiency of ADH (vasopressin) that is secreted by the posterior lobe of the pituitary gland (neurohypophysis)
2. Possible etiology
     a. Trauma to posterior lobe of pituitary gland
     b. Tumor of posterior lobe of pituitary gland
     c. Brain surgery
     d. Head injury

     e. Idiopathic

     f. Meningitis

3. Pathophysiology

     a. Decreased ADH reduces the ability of distal and collecting renal tubules to concentrate urine

     b. Copious, dilute urine and intense thirst result

4. Possible clinical manifestations

     a. Polyuria (greater than 5 liters/day)

     b. Polydipsia (4 to 40 liters/day)

     c. Fatigue

     d. Dehydration

     e. Weight loss

     f. Muscle weakness and pain

     g. Headache

     h. Tachycardia

5. Possible diagnostic test findings

     a. Urine chemistry: specific gravity less than 1.004, osmolality 50 to 200 mOsm/kg

     b. Blood chemistry: decreased ADH by radioimmunoassay

     c. Water deprivation test: inability to concentrate urine

6. Medical management

     a. Diet therapy: regular, with restriction of foods that exert a diuretic effect

     b. I.V. therapy: hydration, electrolyte replacement; heparin lock

     c. Activity: bed rest

     d. Monitoring: VS, UO, CVP, I/O

     e. Laboratory studies: potassium, sodium, BUN, Cr, specific gravity, osmolality

     f. Treatments: Foley catheter

     g. ADH stimulants: chlorpropamide (Diabinese), carbamazepine (Tegretol)

     h. ADH replacement: lypressin (Diapid nasal spray), vasopressin tannate (Pitressin)

     i. Radiation

7. Medical nursing interventions/responsibilities

     a. Maintain diet

     b. Force fluids

     c. Administer I.V. fluids

     d. Assess fluid balance

     e. Maintain patency of Foley catheter

     f. Monitor and record VS, UO, CVP, I/O, specific gravity, laboratory studies

     g. Administer medications

     h. Allay anxiety

     i. Weigh daily

      j. Provide postchemotherapeutic and/or postradiation nursing care: provide skin, mouth, and perineal care; encourage dietary intake; administer antiemetics and antidiarrheals; monitor for bleeding, infection, and electrolyte imbalance; provide rest periods

  8. Patient/family teaching goals; the patient will:
     a. Keep follow-up appointments
     b. Maintain ideal weight
     c. State the action, side effects, and scheduling of medications
     d. Recognize the signs and symptoms of dehydration
     e. Follow dietary recommendations and restrictions
     f. Wear medical identification bracelet
     g. Increase fluid intake in hot weather

  9. Possible medical complications
     a. Dehydration
     b. Dysrhythmias
     c. Hypovolemic shock

10. Possible surgical interventions: none

V. Hyperpituitarism (acromegaly)

  1. Definition: hypersecretion of growth hormone by the anterior pituitary gland (adenohypophysis)

  2. Possible etiology
     a. Prolactin-secreting benign adenomas
     b. Growth-hormone secreting tumors
     c. Cushing's syndrome caused by pituitary dysfunction
     d. LH-, FSH-, or TSH-secreting adenomas
     e. Adrenalectomy
     f. Pregnancy

  3. Pathophysiology
     a. Excessive secretion of growth hormone occurs after epiphyseal closing
     b. Excessive secretion of growth hormone causes overdevelopment of cartilage, bone, soft tissue; thickens skin; enlarges sweat glands, sebaceous glands, and gonads
     c. Growth-hormone-induced hypermetabolism causes hormone alterations

  4. Possible clinical manifestations
     a. Coarse facial features
     b. Enlarged tongue
     c. Protruding jaw
     d. Spiderlike fingers
     e. Wide hands and feet
     f. Weakness
     g. Impotence
     h. Infertility
     i. Thick skin and nails
     j. Diplopia

      k. Cranial nerve palsies
      l. Joint deformities
      m. Pain in joints
      n. Deepening of voice
      o. Diaphoresis
      p. Hirsutism
      q. Headache

5. Possible diagnostic test findings
      a. Insulin tolerance test: hyperglycemia
      b. CT scan: enlarged pituitary
      c. Visual fields: hemianopsia, diplopia
      d. X-rays: thickened long bones and skull
      e. Blood chemistry: increased phosphorus, prolactin, glucose, somatotropin; decreased FSH
      f. Urine chemistry: increased calcium, glucose

6. Medical management
      a. Activity: as tolerated
      b. Monitoring: VS, UO, I/O
      c. Laboratory studies: glucose, potassium, calcium
      d. Radiation therapy
      e. Dopaminergics: levodopa (L-Dopa), bromocrystine mesylate (Parlodel)
      f. Hormones: somatotropin (Somatotropin), ethinyl estadiol (Estinyl), testosterone (Delatestryl), levothyroxine sodium (Synthroid), liothyronine (Cytomel), diethylstilbesterol (Stilbesterol)
      g. Glucocorticoids: cortisone acetate (Cortone), hydrocortisone (Cortef), hydrocortisone sodium succinate (Solu-Cortef)
      h. Ergot alkaloids: methysergide (Sansert)
      i. Mineralocorticoids: fludrocortisone (Florinef)
      j. Cryosurgery
      k. Thermocoagulation
      l. Ultrasound therapy

7. Medical nursing interventions/responsibilities
      a. Assess fluid balance
      b. Monitor and record VS, UO, I/O, urine glucose and ketones, finger sticks, laboratory studies
      c. Administer medications
      d. Encourage ventilation of feelings about change in body image and sexual dysfunction
      e. Maintain activity as tolerated
      f. Provide skin care
      g. Position and support painful joints
      h. Protect from falls
      i. Monitor for infection

  j. Provide postchemotherapeutic and/or postradiation nursing care: provide skin, mouth, and perineal care; encourage dietary intake; administer antiemetics and antidiarrheals; monitor for bleeding, infection, and electrolyte imbalance; provide rest periods

8. Patient/family teaching goals; the patient will:
  a. Keep follow-up appointments
  b. State the action, side effects, and scheduling of medication
  c. Identify and reduce stress
  d. Avoid exposure to people with infections
  e. Alternate rest periods with activity
  f. Monitor self for infection
  g. Promote a safe environment
  h. Maintain a quiet environment
  i. Wear medical indentification bracelet
  j. Carry emergency adrenal hormone replacement drugs

9. Possible medical complications
  a. Blindness
  b. Visual disturbances
  c. Diabetes mellitus
  d. Cushing's syndrome
  e. Hyperthyroidism
  f. Hypertension
  g. CHF
  h. Angina
  i. Cardiomyopathy
  j. Hyperparathyroidism
  k. Renal calculi
  l. Cardiac arrest

10. Possible surgical interventions: hypophysectomy (see page 162)

W. Hypopituitarism (Simmonds' disease)

1. Definition: hypofunction of anterior pituitary gland (adenohypophysis), resulting in insufficient or absent quantities of anterior pituitary gland hormones or target organ hormones

2. Possible etiology
  a. Adenomas or carcinomas of pituitary gland
  b. Postpartum hemorrhage
  c. Head trauma
  d. Necrosis of pituitary gland (Sheehan's syndrome)
  e. Radiation of head
  f. Hypophysectomy
  g. Insufficient hypothalamic releasing factors

3. Pathophysiology
  a. Decreased pituitary function results in decreased amounts of gonadotropic hormone, thyroid-stimulating hormone, and adrenocorticotropic hormone

b. With progressive loss of pituitary function, levels of follicle-stimulating hormone and luteinizing hormone also decrease

4. Possible clinical manifestations
   a. Lethargy
   b. Decreased strength
   c. Decreased tolerance for cold temperatures
   d. Hypothermia
   e. Hypotension
   f. Emaciation
   g. Decreased axillary and pubic hair
   h. Atrophy of gonads and thyroid
   i. Impotence
   j. Weight loss
   k. Pallor
   l. Decreased libido
   m. Amenorrhea
   n. Dry skin
   o. Decreased perspiration
   p. Recurrent infections
   q. Headaches

5. Possible diagnostic test findings
   a. Blood chemistry: decreased cortisol, growth hormone, ACTH, TSH, LH, FSH, glucose, gonadotropins
   b. RAIU: decreased
   c. FBS: decreased glucose
   d. GTT: decreased glucose
   e. Hematology: decreased Hgb, Hct
   f. CT scan: presence of adenohypophyseal tumor
   g. Visual fields: hemianopsia and loss of color vision
   h. Angiography: presence of adenohypophyseal tumor
   i. Urine chemistry: decreased gonadotropins, 17-OHCS, and 17-KS
   j. Skull X-ray: presence of adenohypophyseal tumor

6. Medical management
   g. Diet therapy: high-protein
   a. Activity: as tolerated
   b. Monitoring: VS, UO, I/O, laboratory studies
   c. Radiation therapy
   d. Dopaminergics: levodopa (L-Dopa), bromocrystine mesylate (Parlodel)
   e. Hormones: somatotropin (Somatotropin), ethinyl estadiol (Estinyl), testosterone (Delatestryl), levothyroxine sodium (Synthroid), liothyronine (Cytomel)
   f. Glucocorticoids: cortisone acetate (Cortone), hydrocortisone (Cortef), hydrocortisone sodium succinate (Solu-Cortef)

7. Medical nursing interventions/responsibilities
   a. Maintain diet
   b. Assess fluid balance

  c. Monitor and record VS, UO, I/O, urine glucose and ketones, laboratory studies

  d. Administer medications

  e. Encourage ventilation of feelings about change in body image and sexual dysfunction

  f. Maintain activity as tolerated

  g. Prevent falls

  h. Monitor for infection

  i. Maintain a warm environment

  j. Provide skin care

  k. Allay anxiety

  l. Reinforce need to eat

  m. Provide postchemotherapeutic and/or postradiation nursing care: provide skin, mouth, and perineal care; encourage dietary intake; administer antiemetics and antidiarrheals; monitor for bleeding, infection, and electrolyte imbalance; provide rest periods

8. Patient/family teaching goals; the patient will:

  a. Keep follow-up appointments

  b. Maintain ideal weight

  c. State the action, side effects, and scheduling of medications

  d. Recognize the signs and symptoms of dehydration

  e. Avoid exposure to people with infections

  f. Monitor self for infection

  g. Follow dietary recommendations and restrictions

  h. Promote a safe environment

  i. Maintain a quiet environment

  j. Alternate rest periods with activity

  k. Wear medical identification bracelet

  l. Identify and reduce stressful stimuli

9. Possible medical complications

  a. Death

  b. Hypothyroidism

  c. Adrenal insufficiency

10. Possible surgical interventions

  a. Hypophysectomy (see page 162)

  b. Resection of pituitary gland

Points to Remember

Factors altering the function of the pituitary gland—the "master gland"—affect all hormonal activity.

Changes in secondary sex characteristics and sexual function that accompany diseases of the endocrine system cause embarrassment for patients.

Disturbances in mineralocorticoid and glucocorticoid secretion alter fluid and electrolyte balance.

Anxiety and fear are common responses of patients who have body-image changes associated with endocrine disorders.

A quiet, stress-free environment is important in caring for patients with endocrine disorders.

Glossary

Hirsutism — excessive or unusual placement of hair.

Mineralocorticoid — aldosterone.

Polydipsia — excessive thirst.

Polyphagia — eating abnormally large amounts of food.

Vasopressin — antidiuretic hormone.

Renal System

Learning Objectives

After studying this section, the reader should be able to:

- Describe the psychosocial impact of renal system disorders.

- Differentiate between modifiable and nonmodifiable risk factors in the development of a renal system disorder.

- List three potential and three actual nursing diagnoses for the patient with a renal system disorder.

- Identify the medical and surgical nursing interventions/responsibilities for the patient with a renal system disorder.

- Write three teaching goals for the patient with a renal system disorder.

VI. Renal System

A. Anatomy and physiology

1. Kidneys
   a. Bean-shaped organs
   b. Components: cortex, medulla, renal pelvis, and nephron
   c. Cortex: outer layer of kidney, containing glomeruli, proximal tubules of nephron, and distal tubules of nephron
   d. Medulla: inner layer of kidney, containing loops of Henle and collecting tubules
   e. Renal pelvis: collects urine from calices
   f. Nephron: functional unit of kidney composed of Bowman's capsule, glomerulus, and renal tubule
   g. Renal tubule: consists of proximal convoluted, loop of Henle, distal convoluted and collecting segments
2. Ureter
   a. This tubule extends from renal pelvis to bladder floor
   b. It transports urine from kidney to bladder
   c. Ureterovesical sphincter prevents reflux of urine from bladder into ureter
3. Bladder
   a. Muscular, distendable sack that stores urine
   b. Total capacity approximately 1 liter
4. Urethra
   a. This tubule extends from the bladder to the urinary meatus
   b. It transports urine from bladder to urinary meatus
5. Urine formation
   a. Blood from renal artery is filtrated across the glomerular capillary membrane in Bowman's capsule
   b. Filtration requires adequate intravascular volume and adequate cardiac output
   c. Composition of formed filtrate is similar to blood plasma without proteins
   d. As formed filtrate moves through the tubules of the nephron, electrolytes, water, glucose, amino acids, ammonia, and bicarbonate are reabsorbed and secreted
   e. Antidiuretic hormone (ADH) and aldosterone control the reabsorption of water and electrolytes
6. Blood pressure control
   a. Regulation of fluid volume by the kidney affects blood pressure
   b. Renin-angiotensin system is activated by decreased blood pressure
7. Prostate gland
   a. This fibrous capsule is connected to and surrounds male urethra
   b. It contains ducts that secrete the alkaline portion of seminal fluid and open into the prostatic portion of the urethra

B. Physical assessment findings
1. Subjective data that often accompany renal disorders
   a. Change in pattern of urination: frequency, nocturia, hesitancy, urgency, dribbling, incontinence, and retention
   b. Change in appearance of urine: dilute, concentrated, hematuria, and pyuria
   c. Dysuria
   d. Pain
   e. Chills and fever
2. Objective data to evaluate in renal disorders
   a. Urine output: polyuria, oliguria, and anuria
   b. Specific gravity
   c. Hematuria
   d. Urine pH
   e. Periorbital and peripheral edema
   f. Bladder distention
   g. Skin coloring
   h. Comparison of total intake and output (I/O)
   i. Muscle tremors
   j. Pattern and character of respirations
   k. Size of prostate gland
   l. Temperature

C. Diagnostic tests and procedures used to evaluate renal disorders
1. Urinalysis
   a. Definition/purpose: microscopic examination of the urine for color, appearance, pH, specific gravity, protein, glucose, ketones, red blood cells (RBC), white blood cells (WBC), and casts
   b. Nursing interventions/responsibilites: wash perineal area; obtain first morning specimen
2. Urine culture and sensitivity
   a. Definition/purpose: microscopic examination of the urine for bacteria
   b. Nursing interventions/responsibilities: clean perineal area and urinary meatus with bacteriostatic solution; collect midstream sample in sterile container
3. 24-hour urine collection
   a. Definition/purpose: quantitative laboratory analysis of urine collected over 24 hours to determine kidney function
   b. Nursing interventions/responsibilities: instruct patient to void and note time (collection starts with the next voiding); place urine container on ice; measure each voided urine; instruct patient to void at end of 24-hour period; note medications that might alter tests results
4. Blood chemistry
   a. Definition/purpose: laboratory analysis of blood sample for potassium, sodium, calcium, phosphorus, glucose, bicarbonate, blood urea nitrogen (BUN), creatinine (Cr), protein, albumin, and osmolality

    b. Nursing interventions/responsibilities: before procedure, withhold food and fluids, as ordered; after procedure, monitor site for bleeding

5. Kidneys, ureters, bladder (KUB) X-ray
    a. Definition/purpose: radiographic picture of the kidneys, ureters, and bladder
    b. Nursing interventions/responsibilities: schedule before other examinations requiring contrast medium; remove metallic belts

6. I.V. pyelogram (IVP)
    a. Definition/purpose: fluoroscopic examination of kidneys, ureters, and bladder after injection of a radiopaque dye
    b. Nursing interventions/responsibilities: before procedure, assess allergies to iodine, seafood, or radiopaque dyes; withhold food and fluids after midnight; administer laxatives as ordered; instruct patient he may feel flushing of the face and throat irritation; after procedure, instruct patient to drink at least 1 liter of fluids; assess insertion site for bleeding

7. Cystoscopy
    a. Definition/purpose: direct visualization of the bladder using a cystoscope
    b. Nursing interventions/responsibilities: before procedure, withhold food and fluids; allay anxiety; obtain written, informed consent; administer enemas and medications as ordered; after procedure, administer analgesics and sitz baths as ordered; monitor I/O and vital signs (VS); assess urine for clots; force fluids

8. Renal angiography
    a. Definition/purpose: radiographic examination of the renal arterial supply after injection of radiopaque dye through a catheter
    b. Nursing interventions/responsibilities: before procedure, allay anxiety; instruct patient he may feel burning after dye is injected; obtain written, informed consent; withhold food and fluids after midnight; instruct patient to void immediately before procedure; administer enemas as ordered; after procedure, assess VS and peripheral pulses; inspect catheter insertion site for bleeding; force fluids

9. Renal scan
    a. Definition/purpose: visual imaging of blood flow distribution to kidneys after I.V. injection of a radioisotope
    b. Nursing interventions/responsibilities: before procedure, administer Lugol's solution as ordered; after procedure, continue the administration of Lugol's solution as ordered; wear gloves when caring for incontinent patients and double-bag linens

10. Renal biopsy
    a. Definition/purpose: percutaneous removal of small amount of renal tissue for histologic evaluation
    b. Nursing interventions/responsibilities: before procedure, assess baseline clotting studies and VS, withhold food and fluids after midnight; obtain written, informed consent; after procedure, monitor VS, hemoglobin (Hgb) and hematocrit (Hct); assess biopsy site for bleeding

11. Cystourethrogram
    a. Definition/purpose: visualization of bladder and ureters after insertion of a catheter and introduction of dye
    b. Nursing interventions/responsibilities: before procedure, allay anxiety; advise patient that he will be asked to void during the procedure; after procedure, monitor voiding
12. Cystometrogram
    a. Definition/purpose: graphic recording of the pressures exerted at varying phases of filling of the urinary bladder
    b. Nursing interventions/responsibilities: before procedure, allay anxiety; advise the patient he will be asked to void during the procedure; after procedure, monitor voiding
13. Hematologic studies
    a. Definition/purpose: laboratory analysis of blood sample for WBC, RBC, erythrocyte sedimentation rate (ESR), platelets, prothrombin time (PT), partial thromboplastin time (PTT), Hgb, and Hct
    b. Nursing interventions/responsibilities: assess site for bleeding

D. **Possible psychosocial impact of renal disorders**
    1. Developmental impact
       a. Body image changes
       b. Feeling of lack of control over body function
       c. Fear of rejection
       d. Embarrassment from change in body function and structure
       e. Decreased self-esteem
    2. Economic impact
       a. Cost of renal dialysis and transplantation
       b. Cost of hospitalizations and follow-up care
       c. Cost of medications
       d. Cost of special diet
       e. Disruption of employment
    3. Occupational and recreational impact
       a. Restrictions in physical activity
       b. Change in leisure activity
    4. Social impact
       a. Change in eating patterns
       b. Social isolation
       c. Change in elimination patterns and modes
       d. Change in sexual function

E. **Possible risk factors for development of renal disorders**
    1. Modifiable risk factors
       a. Diet: high-sodium, high-calcium
       b. Exposure to chemical and environmental pollutants
       c. Smoking
       d. Contact sports

2. Nonmodifiable risk factors
   a. Culturally based reluctance to discuss hygiene and health habits
   b. History of renal dysfunction
   c. History of hypertension
   d. Aging process
   e. Family history of renal disease

F. **Possible nursing diagnoses for the patient with renal disorders**
   1. Actual nursing diagnoses
      a. Fluid volume deficit
      b. Alteration in fluid volume: excess
      c. Alteration in pattern of urinary elimination
      d. Alteration in comfort: pain
      e. Sexual dysfunction
      f. Disturbance in self-concept: body image
      g. Disturbance in self-concept: self-esteem
   2. Potential nursing diagnoses
      a. Impairment of skin integrity
      b. Noncompliance
      c. Activity intolerance
      d. Anticipatory grieving
      e. Impaired gas exchange

G. **Surgical intervention: kidney transplant**
   1. Definition: transplant of kidney from donor to a person who requires dialysis for end stage renal disease
   2. Preoperative surgical nursing interventions/responsibilities
      a. Complete patient and family preoperative teaching: assess understanding of surgical procedure; explain operating room (OR), recovery room (RR), preoperative and postoperative routine; demonstrate postoperative turning, coughing, and deep breathing (TCDB), splinting, leg exercises, and range-of-motion exercises (ROM); explain postoperative need for drainage tubes, surgical dressings, oxygen therapy, I.V. therapy, and pain control
      b. Complete preoperative check list
      c. Administer preoperative medications
      d. Allay patient and family anxiety about surgery
      e. Document patient history and physical assessment data base
      f. Verify histocompatability tests
      g. Administer immunosuppressive drugs for 2 days prior to transplant
      h. Maintain protective isolation
      i. Administer transfusion therapy
      j. Administer I.V. therapy
      k. Monitor urinary output (UO)
      l. Verify that hemodialysis was completed 24 hours before transplant

3. Postoperative surgical nursing interventions/responsibilities
   a. Assess cardiac and respiratory status and fluid balance
   b. Assess pain and administer postoperative analgesic
   c. Progress diet as tolerated
   d. Administer I.V. fluids
   e. Allay anxiety
   f. Assess surgical dressing and change as directed
   g. Reinforce TCDB and splinting of incision
   h. Maintain semi-Fowler position
   i. Assess for return of peristalsis
   j. Provide pulmonary toilet: incentive spirometry, intermittent positive pressure breathing (IPPB)
   k. Maintain activity: as tolerated, progressive ambulation
   l. Monitor and record VS, UO, I/O, central venous pressure (CVP), laboratory studies, urine for blood, EKG, specific gravity, daily weight
   m. Monitor and maintain position and patency of drainage tubes: Foley, nasogastric (NG), wound drainage
   n. Precautions: protective
   o. Encourage ventilation of feelings about chronicity of illness, fear of dying
   p. Administer antifungals
   q. Administer immunosuppressive agents
   r. Administer corticosteroids
   s. Assess for organ rejection
   t. Monitor for infection
   u. Provide mouth and skin care
   v. Administer antibiotics
   w. Administer antilymphocytic globulin (ALG) and antithymocytic globulin (ATG)
   x. Prepare for hemodialysis
   y. Avoid prolonged periods of sitting
4. Possible surgical complications
   a. Renal graft rejection
   b. Gastrointestinal hemorrhage
   c. Acute renal failure
   d. Bladder and ureter fistulas
   e. Candidiasis of mouth
   f. Hypertension
   g. Cerebrovascular accident (CVA)
   h. Gastric ulcer
   i. Liver failure
5. Patient/family postoperative teaching goals; the patient will:
   a. Keep follow-up appointments
   b. Stop smoking
   c. Maintain ideal weight
   d. State the action, side effects, and scheduling of medications

e. Recognize the signs and symptoms of infection and rejection
f. Avoid contact sports
g. Complete daily incision care
h. Adhere to low-sodium and low-protein diet
i. Avoid exposure to people with infections
j. Monitor stool for occult blood
k. Monitor self for infection

H. Surgical intervention: kidney surgery

1. Definition
   a. Nephrectomy: surgical removal of the entire kidney
   b. Lithotomy: surgical removal of renal calculi
2. Preoperative surgical nursing interventions/responsibilities
   a. Complete patient and family preoperative teaching: assess understanding of surgical procedure; explain OR, RR, preoperative and postoperative routine; demonstrate postoperative TCDB, splinting, leg exercises, and ROM; explain postoperative need for drainage tubes, surgical dressings, oxygen therapy, I.V. therapy, and pain control
   b. Complete preoperative check list
   c. Administer preoperative medications
   d. Allay patient and family anxiety about surgery
   e. Document patient history and physical assessment data base
   f. Administer antibiotics
3. Postoperative surgical nursing interventions/responsibilities
   a. Assess cardiac, respiratory, and neurologic status and fluid balance
   b. Assess pain and administer postoperative analgesic
   c. Progress diet as tolerated with increased fluids
   d. Administer I.V. fluids, transfusion therapy, and IVH
   e. Allay anxiety
   f. Assess surgical dressing and change as directed
   g. Reinforce TCDB and splinting of incision
   h. Maintain semi-Fowler position
   i. Assess for return of peristalsis
   j. Provide pulmonary toilet: incentive spirometry
   k. Maintain activity: as tolerated, active and passive ROM, progressive ambulation
   l. Monitor and record VS, UO, I/O, CVP, laboratory studies, urine for blood, daily weight, specific gravity
   m. Monitor and maintain position and patency of drainage tubes: NG, Foley, wound drainage, nephrostomy, suprapubic, ureteral
   n. Encourage ventilation of feelings about change in body image and fear of dying
   o. Administer antibiotics
   p. Administer stool softeners
   q. Do not irrigate or manipulate nephrostomy tube
   r. Apply antiembolitic stockings

    4. Possible surgical complications
      a. Hemorrhage
      b. Atelectasis
      c. Pneumothorax
      d. Pneumonia
      e. Paralytic ileus
    5. Patient/family postoperative teaching goals; the patient will:
      a. Keep follow-up appointments
      b. State the action, side effects, and scheduling of medications
      c. Recognize the signs and symptoms of infection and renal failure
      d. Complete daily incision care
      e. Avoid use of over-the-counter medications
      f. Increase fluid intake using cranberry juice
      g. Avoid lifting, straining, horseback riding, and contact sports
      h. Void frequently

I. Surgical intervention: prostate surgery
    1. Definition
      a. Transurethral resection of prostate (TURP): insertion of resectoscope into urethra to excise prostatic tissue
      b. Suprapubic prostatectomy: low abdominal incision into the bladder to the anterior aspect of the prostate to remove large tumors of the prostate
      c. Retropubic prostatectomy: low midline incision below the bladder into prostatic capsule to remove a mass in the pelvic area
      d. Perineal prostatectomy: incision through perineum to remove the prostate and surrounding tissue
    2. Preoperative surgical nursing interventions/responsibilities
      a. Complete patient and family preoperative teaching: assess understanding of surgical procedure; explain OR, RR, preoperative and postoperative routine; demonstrate postoperative TCDB, splinting, leg exercises, and ROM; explain postoperative need for drainage tubes, surgical dressings, oxygen therpy, I.V. therapy, and pain control
      b. Complete preoperative check list
      c. Administer preoperative medications
      d. Allay patient and family anxiety about surgery
      e. Document patient history and physical assessment data base
      f. Administer antibiotics
    3. Postoperative surgical nursing interventions/responsibilities
      a. Assess cardiac and respiratory status and fluid balance
      b. Assess pain and administer postoperative analgesic
      c. Progress high-protein, high-fiber, acid/ash diet as tolerated with increased fluids
      d. Administer I.V. fluids
      e. Allay anxiety
      f. Assess surgical dressing and change as directed
      g. Reinforce TCDB and splinting of incision

    h. Maintain semi-Fowler position

    i. Assess for return of peristalsis

    j. Provide pulmonary toilet: incentive spirometry

    k. Maintain activity: as tolerated, progressive ambulation

    l. Monitor and record VS, UO, I/O, laboratory studies, urine for blood, stool counts

    m. Monitor and maintain position and patency of drainage tubes: NG, Foley, wound drainage, suprapubic

    n. Encourage ventilation of feelings about change in body image and fear of sexual dysfunction

    o. Administer stool softeners

    p. Maintain closed continuous bladder irrigation

    q. Administer antibiotics

    r. Provide treatments: sitz baths

    s. Administer anticholinergics

    t. Administer antispasmodics

    u. Avoid rectal temperatures and enemas

    v. Administer urinary antiseptics

    w. Monitor urinary patterns after removal of catheters

4. Possible surgical complications

    a. Hemorrhage

    b. Shock

    c. Infection

    d. Epididymitis

    e. Impotence

5. Patient/family postoperative teaching goals; the patient will:

    a. Keep follow-up appointments

    b. Stop smoking

    c. State the action, side effects, and scheduling of medications

    d. Recognize the signs and symptoms of infection, bleeding, and urinary tract obstruction

    e. Complete daily incision care

    f. Avoid use of over-the-counter medications

    g. Avoid Valsalva's maneuver, sitting for prolonged periods in the car, lifting, vigorous exercise

    h. Increase fluid intake

    i. Complete daily perineal strengthening exercises

    j. Avoid alcohol and caffeine

J. Surgical intervention: urinary diversion

1. Definition

    a. Ureterosigmoidostomy: ureters are excised from bladder and implanted into sigmoid colon; urine flows through colon and is excreted through rectum

    b. Nephrostomy: percutaneous insertion of catheter into kidney

    c. Ileal conduit: ureters are implanted into a segment of the ileum that has been resected from the intestinal tract with the formation of an abdominal stoma

    d. Cutaneous ureterostomy: ureters are excised from the bladder and brought through the abdominal wall to create a stoma

2. Preoperative surgical nursing interventions/responsibilities

    a. Complete patient and family preoperative teaching: assess understanding of surgical procedure; explain OR, RR, preoperative and postoperative routine; demonstrate postoperative TCDB, splinting, leg exercises, and ROM; explain postoperative need for drainage tubes, surgical dressings, oxygen therapy, I.V. therapy, and pain control

    b. Complete preoperative check list

    c. Administer preoperative medications

    d. Allay patient and family anxiety about surgery

    e. Document patient history and physical assessment data base

    f. Administer bowel preparation

3. Postoperative surgical nursing interventions/responsibilities

    a. Assess renal status and fluid balance

    b. Assess pain and administer postoperative analgesic

    c. Progress acid/ash diet as tolerated with increased fluids; avoid milk and dairy products

    d. Administer I.V. fluids

    e. Allay anxiety

    f. Assess surgical dressing and change as directed

    g. Reinforce TCDB and splinting of incision

    h. Maintain semi-Fowler position

    i. Assess for return of peristalsis

    j. Provide pulmonary toilet: incentive spirometry

    k. Maintain activity: as tolerated, progressive ambulation

    l. Monitor and record VS, UO, I/O, laboratory studies, daily weights, specific gravity

    m. Monitor and maintain position and patency of drainage tubes: NG, Foley, wound drainage

    n. Encourage ventilation of feelings about change in body image, embarrassment, and sexual dysfunction

    o. Administer antibiotics

    p. Administer antispasmodics

    q. Apply and change specialized appliances: ostomy bags

    r. Provide skin care, particularly around stoma

    s. Apply antiembolitic stockings

4. Possible surgical complications

    a. Chronic renal failure

    b. Infection

    c. Urinary and rectal fistulas

    d. Hemorrhage

    e. Peritonitis

f. Ureteral obstruction
g. Stomal stenosis
h. Bowel obstruction
i. Renal calculi
5. Patient/family postoperative teaching goals; the patient will:
   a. Keep follow-up appointments
   b. State the action, side effects, and scheduling of medications
   c. Recognize the signs and symptoms of infection and stomal stenosis
   d. Complete daily stoma and skin care
   e. Use specialized appliances: ostomy bags, face plates, and leg bags
   f. Increase fluid intake
   g. Follow dietary recommendations and restrictions
   h. Avoid enemas and laxatives
   i. Empty urinary diversion appliances frequently

K. Cystitis
1. Definition: inflammation of the urinary bladder related to a superficial infection that does not extend to the bladder mucosa
2. Possible etiology
   a. Stagnation of urine in bladder
   b. Obstruction of urethra
   c. Sexual intercourse
   d. Incorrect aseptic technique during catheterization
   e. Incorrect perineal care
   f. Kidney infection
   g. Radiation
   h. Diabetes mellitus
   i. Pregnancy
3. Pathophysiology
   a. Bacterial infection from secondary source spreads to bladder, causing inflammatory response
   b. Cell destruction from trauma to the bladder wall, particularly the trigone area, initiates an acute inflammatory reaction
4. Possible clinical manifestations
   a. Frequency of urination
   b. Urgency of urination
   c. Burning or pain on urination
   d. Lower abdominal discomfort
   e. Dark, odoriferous urine
   f. Flank tenderness or suprapubic pain
   g. Nocturia
   h. Low-grade fever
   i. Urge to bear down on urination
   j. Dysuria
   k. Dribbling

5. Possible diagnostic test findings
   a. Urine culture and sensitivity: positive identification of organisms (*E. coli, P. vulgaris, S. faecalis*)
   b. Urine chemistry: hematuria, pyuria; increased protein, leukocytes, specific gravity
   c. Cystoscopy: presence of obstruction or deformity
6. Medical management
   a. Diet therapy: acid/ash, with increased intake of fluids and vitamin C
   b. Activity: as tolerated
   c. Monitoring: VS, UO, I/O
   d. Laboratory studies: specific gravity, urine culture and sensitivity
   e. Treatments: sitz baths
   f. Antibiotics: trimethoprim and sulfamethoxazole (Bactrim), cephalexin (Keflex)
   g. Analgesics: oxycodone hydrochloride (Tylox)
   h. Urinary antiseptics: phenazopyridine (Pyridium)
   i. Antipyretics: acetaminophen (Tylenol)
7. Medical nursing interventions/responsibilities
   a. Maintain diet
   b. Force fluids to 3,000 ml/day using cranberry or orange juice
   c. Assess renal status
   d. Monitor and record VS, UO, I/O, laboratory studies
   e. Administer medications
   f. Allay anxiety
   g. Maintain treatments: sitz baths, perineal care
   h. Encouraging voiding every 2 to 3 hours
8. Patient/family teaching goals; the patient will:
   a. Keep follow-up appointments
   b. Stop smoking
   c. State the action, side effects, and scheduling of medications
   d. Recognize the signs and symptoms of recurrent infection
   e. Avoid coffee, tea, alcohol, and cola
   f. Increase fluid intake to 3,000 ml/day using orange juice and cranberry juice
   g. Void every 2 to 3 hours and after intercourse
   h. Perform perineal care correctly
   i. Avoid bubble baths, vaginal deodorants, and tub baths
9. Possible medical complications
   a. Chronic cystitis
   b. Urethritis
   c. Pyelonephritis
10. Possible surgical interventions: none

L. Glomerulonephritis
1. Definition: Inflammation of capillary loops in the glomeruli of the kidney
2. Possible etiology
   a. Injected serum proteins
   b. Systemic lupus erythematosus
   c. Group A beta-hemolytic streptococcal infection
3. Pathophysiology
   a. Antigen-antibody complexes are filtered and trapped within the glomeruli, causing inflammation
   b. Inflammation occludes the glomeruli, causing decreased glomerular filtration and retention of protein wastes and electrolytes
4. Possible clinical manifestations
   a. Bradycardia
   b. Pharyngitis and tonsillitis
   c. Peripheral and periorbital edema
   d. Lethargy and malaise
   e. Anorexia
   f. Elevated temperature
   g. Hypertension
   h. Tea-colored urine
   i. Flank pain
   j. Dyspnea
   k. Visual disturbances
   l. Dizziness
   m. Oliguria
   n. Convulsions
   o. Weight loss
   p. Dehydration
5. Possible diagnostic test findings
   a. Urine chemistry: increased RBC, WBC, protein, casts, specific gravity
   b. Blood chemistry: increased BUN, Cr; decreased protein, creatine clearance, C-reactive protein, albumin
   c. Hematology: decreased Hgb, Hct; increased ESR
   d. Renal biopsy: inflammation of glomerular capillaries
6. Medical management
   a. Diet therapy: high-carbohydrate, high-vitamin, with restricted intake of sodium, protein, potassium, and fluids
   b. I.V. therapy: heparin lock
   c. Activity: bed rest
   d. Monitoring: VS, UO, I/O, EKG
   e. Laboratory studies: BUN, Cr, specific gravity, sodium, potassium, glucose, Hgb, Hct
   f. Antibiotics: penicillin (PenVee K), ampicillin (Omnipen)
   g. Antihypertensives: diazoxide (Hyperstat), hydralazine hydrochloride (Apresoline)

   h. Cardioglycoside: digoxin (Lanoxin)
   i. Immunosuppressants: cyclophosphamide (Cytoxan), azathioprine (Imuran)
   j. Antacids: magnesium and aluminum hydroxide (Maalox), aluminum hydroxide gel (Alternagel)
   k. Corticosteroids: prednisone (Deltasone)
   l. Diuretics: chlorthalidone (Hygroton), furosemide (Lasix)
   m. Peritoneal dialysis and hemodialysis
   n. Anticoagulants: warfarin sodium (Coumadin), sodium heparin (Lipo-Hepin)
   o. Precautions: seizure
7. Medical nursing interventions/responsibilities
   a. Maintain diet
   b. Restrict fluids
   c. Reinforce TCDB
   d. Assess renal, respiratory, cardiovascular, neurologic status and fluid balance
   e. Monitor and record VS, UO, I/O, EKG, laboratory studies, urine glucose and ketones, hematuria, weight, specific gravity
   f. Administer medications
   g. Encourage ventilation of feelings about change in body image
   h. Maintain seizure precautions
   i. Protect from falls
   j. Monitor for bleeding and infection
   k. Provide skin and mouth care
8. Patient/family teaching goals; the patient will:
   a. Keep follow-up appointments
   b. Stop smoking
   c. Maintain ideal weight
   d. State the action, side effects, and scheduling of medications
   e. Recognize the signs and symptoms of renal failure
   f. Avoid exposure to people with infections
   g. Alternate rest periods with activity
   h. Monitor self for infection
   i. Follow dietary recommendations and restrictions
9. Possible medical complications
   a. Metabolic acidosis
   b. Chronic renal failure
   c. Hypertensive encephalopathy
   d. Congestive heart failure (CHF)
   e. Nephrotic syndrome
   f. Pulmonary edema
10. Possible surgical interventions: none

M. Pyelonephritis
1. Definition: inflammation of renal pelvis
2. Possible etiology
   a. Enteric bacteria
   b. Ureterovesical reflux
   c. Urinary tract obstruction
   d. Pregnancy
   e. Trauma
   f. Urinary tract infection
   g. Incorrect aseptic technique
   h. Diabetes mellitus
   i. Staphylococcal or streptococcal infections
3. Pathophysiology
   a. Bacterial infection from secondary source spreads to renal pelvis, causing inflammatory response
   b. Cell destruction from trauma to the renal pelvis initiates an inflammatory reaction
4. Possible clinical manifestations
   a. Elevated temperature
   b. Chills
   c. Nausea and vomiting
   d. Flank pain
   e. Chronic fatigue
   f. Bladder irritability
   g. Hypertension
   h. Dysuria
   i. Burning on urination
   j. Frequency of urination
   k. Urgency of urination
   l. Headache
   m. Anorexia
   n. Weight loss
   o. Odoriferous, concentrated urine
5. Possible diagnostic test findings
   a. IVP: atrophy, blockage, or deformity of kidney
   b. Urine culture and sensitivity: presence of bacteria
   c. Urine chemistry: pyuria, hematuria; presence of leukocytes, WBCs, and casts; specific gravity greater than 1.025; albuminuria
   d. Hematology: increased WBC
   e. 24-hour urine collection: decreased Cr clearance
6. Medical management
   a. Diet therapy: soft, high-calorie, low-protein
   b. I.V. therapy: heparin lock
   c. Activity: as tolerated
   d. Monitoring: VS, UO, I/O, urine pH, specific gravity
   e. Laboratory studies: WBC, urine protein, urine culture and sensitivity

      f. Treatments: warm, moist compresses to flank
      g. Fluid intake: 3,000 ml/day
      h. Analgesics: meperidine hydrochloride (Demerol)
      i. Antibiotics: cefazolin (Ancef), cefoxitin (Mefoxin), trimethoprim and sufamethoxazole (Bactrim)
      j. Urinary antiseptics: phenazopyridine (Pyridium)
      k. Antiemetics: prochlorperazine (Compazine)
      l. Alkalinizers: potassium acetate, sodium bicarbonate
      m. Sedatives: phenobarbital (Luminal)
      n. Peritoneal dialysis and hemodialysis

7. Medical nursing interventions/responsibilities
      a. Maintain diet
      b. Force fluids to 3,000 ml/day
      c. Assess renal status and fluid balance
      d. Monitor and record VS, UO, I/O, laboratory studies, daily weights, specific gravity, urine for blood, protein, pH
      e. Administer medications
      f. Allay anxiety
      g. Maintain treatments: hot, moist compresses; warm baths
      h. Prevent chilling
      i. Provide rest periods
      j. Provide skin, mouth, and perineal care
      k. Encourage frequent voiding

8. Patient/family teaching goals; the patient will:
      a. Keep follow-up appointments
      b. State the action, side effects, and scheduling of medications
      c. Recognize the signs and symptoms of urinary tract infection
      d. Alternate rest periods with activity
      e. Follow dietary recommendations and restrictions
      f. Void frequently

9. Possible medical complications
      a. Chronic renal failure
      b. Hypertension
      c. Septicemia

10. Possible surgical interventions: none

N. Urolithiasis

1. Definition: Presence of stones in kidney, ureters, or bladder
2. Possible etiology
      a. Diet high in calcium, vitamin D, milk, protein, oxalate, alkali
      b. Gout
      c. Hyperparathyroidism
      d. Urinary tract infection
      e. Urinary stasis
      f. Dehydration
      g. Idiopathic

     h. Immobility
     i. Genetics
     j. Hypercalcemia
     k. Urinary tract obstruction
     l. Leukemia
     m. Polycythemia vera
     n. Chemotherapy

3. Pathophysiology
     a. Crystalline substances that normally are dissolved and excreted in the urine form precipitates
     b. Stones are composed of calcium phosphate, oxalate, or uric acid

4. Possible clinical manifestations
     a. Flank pain
     b. Costovertebral tenderness
     c. Cool, moist skin
     d. Renal colic
     e. Frequency of urination
     f. Urgency of urination
     g. Diaphoresis
     h. Chills and fever
     i. Pallor
     j. Nausea and vomiting
     k. Syncope
     l. Dysuria

5. Possible diagnostic test findings
     a. KUB: presence of stones
     b. IVP: presence of stones
     c. Urine chemistry: pyuria, proteinuria, hematuria, presence of WBCs, increased specific gravity
     d. Cystoscopy: visualization of stones
     e. 24-hour urine collection: increased uric acid, oxalate, calcium, phosphorus, Cr
     f. Blood chemistry: increased calcium, phosphorus, Cr, BUN, uric acid, protein, alkaline phosphatase

6. Medical management
     a. Diet therapy: acid/ash, with limited intake of calcium and milk products, for calcium stones; alkaline-ash, with limited intake of foods high in oxalate (cola, tea), for oxalate stones; alkaline/ash, with limited intake of foods high in purine, for uric acid stones
     b. IV therapy: heparin lock
     c. Activity: as tolerated
     d. Monitoring: VS, UO, I/O, urine pH
     e. Laboratory studies: Cr, BUN, phosphorus, calcium, protein
     f. Treatments: strain urine, moist heat to flank, hot baths
     g. Force fluids to 3,000 ml/day
     h. Antigout agents: sulfinpyrazone (Anturane)

      i. Analgesics: meperidine hydrochloride (Demerol)
      j. Antibiotics: cefazolin (Ancef), cefoxitin (Mefoxin)
      k. Antiemetics: prochlorperazine (Compazine)
      l. Acidifiers: ammonium chloride, methenamine mandelate (Mandelamine)
      m. Alkalinizers: potassium acetate, sodium bicarbonate
      n. Chemolysis
      o. Electrohydraulic lithotrypsy
      p. Ultrasonic lithotrypsy
      q. Laser impulse

7. Medical nursing interventions/responsibilities
      a. Maintain diet
      b. Force fluids to 3,000 ml/day
      c. Assess renal status
      d. Monitor and record VS, UO, I/O, daily weights, specific gravity, laboratory studies, urine pH
      e. Administer medications
      f. Allay anxiety
      g. Maintain treatments: strain urine, warm baths, warm soaks to flank
      h. Assess pain

8. Patient/family teaching goals; the patient will:
      a. Keep follow-up appointments
      b. Maintain regular exercise program
      c. State the action, side effects, and scheduling of medications
      d. Recognize the signs and symptoms of urinary tract infection
      e. Alternate rest periods with activity
      f. Monitor self for infection
      g. Follow dietary recommendations and restrictions
      h. Increase fluid intake, especially during hot weather, illness, exercise
      i. Void when urge is felt
      j. Test urine pH
      k. Increase fluids at night and void frequently

9. Possible medical complications
      a. Chronic urinary tract infection
      b. Renal obstruction
      c. Ureterovesical reflux
      d. Hydronephrosis
      e. Pyelonephritis

10. Possible surgical interventions: lithotomy (see page 201)

O. Acute renal failure

1. Definition: sudden inability of the kidneys to regulate fluid and electrolyte balance and remove toxic products from the body
2. Possible etiology
      a. CHF
      b. Cardiogenic shock
      c. Hemorrhage

     d. Burns
     e. Septicemia
     f. Hypotension
     g. Acute tubular necrosis
     h. Acute vasoconstriction
     i. Endocarditis
     j. Malignant hypertension
     k. Diabetes mellitus
     l. Dehydration
     m. Tumor
     n. Blood transfusion reaction
     o. Cardiopulmonary bypass
     p. Nephrotoxins: antibiotics, X-ray dyes, pesticides, anesthetics
     q. Renal calculi
     r. Benign prostatic hypertrophy
     s. Acute glomerulonephritis
     t. Trauma
     u. Congenital deformity
     v. Anaphylaxis
     w. Collagen diseases

3. Pathophysiology
     a. Decreased perfusion of the kidney results in decreased blood flow and glomerular filtrate, ischemia, and oliguria
     b. Damaged nephrons are unable to absorb and secrete water, electrolytes, glucose, amino acids, ammonia, and bicarbonate
     c. Disorder may progress from anuric or oliguric phase through diuretic phase to convalescence phase to recovery of function
     d. Disorder may develop into chronic renal failure

4. Possible clinical manifestions
     a. Urine output less than 400 ml/day for 1 to 2 weeks followed by diuresis (3 to 5 liters/day) for 2 to 3 weeks
     b. Lethargy
     c. Drowsiness
     d. Stupor
     e. Coma
     f. Irritability
     g. Headache
     h. Costovertebral pain
     i. Circumoral numbness
     j. Tingling extremities
     k. Anorexia
     l. Restlessness
     m. Weight gain
     n. Nausea and vomiting
     o. Pallor
     p. Epistaxis

q. Ecchymosis
r. Diarrhea or constipation
s. Stomatitis
t. Thick, tenacious sputum
5. Possible diagnostic test findings
   a. Blood chemistry: increased potassium, phosphorus, magnesium, BUN, Cr, uric acid; decreased calcium, CO_2, sodium
   b. Hematology: decreased Hgb, Hct, erythrocytes; increased prothrombin time (PT), partial thromboplastin time (PTT)
   c. Urine chemistry: albuminuria, proteinuria, increased sodium; presence of casts, RBCs, and WBCs; specific gravity greater than 1.025, then fixed at less than 1.010
   d. IVP: decreased renal perfusion and function
   e. Phenolsulfonphthalein (PSF): decreased
   f. Arterial blood gases (ABGs): metabolic acidosis
6. Medical management
   a. Diet therapy: low-protein, increased-carbohydrate, moderate-fat, and moderate-calorie with potassium, sodium and phosphorus intake regulated according to serum levels
   b. I.V. therapy: electrolyte replacement, heparin lock
   c. Position: semi-Fowler
   d. Activity: bed rest, active and passive ROM, isometric exercises
   e. Monitoring: VS, UO, I/O, EKG, CVP
   f. Laboratory studies: BUN, Cr, phosphorus, calcium, potassium, sodium, Hgb, Hct, specific gravity
   g. Nutritional support: IVH
   h. Treatments: Foley catheter, incentive spirometry, cooling blanket
   i. Fluids: restrict intake to amount needed to replace fluid loss
   j. Transfusion therapy: packed red blood cells (PRBC)
   k. Antibiotics: cefazolin (Ancef), cefoxitin (Mefoxin)
   l. Analgesics: oxycodone hydrochloride (Tylox)
   m. Diuretics: furosemide (Lasix), mannitol (Osmitrol)
   n. Antacids: aluminum hydroxide gel (Alternagel)
   o. Antiemetics: prochlorperazine (Compazine)
   p. Cation exchange resins: sodium polystyrene sulfonate (Kayexalate)
   q. Chelating agents: dimercaprol (BAL)
   r. Beta adrenergics: dopamine hydrochloride (Intropin)
   s. Anticonvulsants: phenytoin sodium (Dilantin)
   t. Peritoneal dialysis and hemodialysis
   u. Antipyretics: acetaminophen (Tylenol)
   v. Precautions: seizure
   w. Alkalinizing agent: sodium bicarbonate
7. Medical nursing interventions/responsibilities
   a. Maintain diet
   b. Restrict fluids
   c. Administer I.V. fluids

     d. Assess fluid balance, respiratory, cardiovascular, and neurologic status

     e. Maintain semi-Fowler position

     f. Monitor and record VS, UO, I/O, CVP, daily weight, specific gravity, laboratory studies, stool for occult blood, urine glucose and ketones

     g. Administer IVH

     h. Administer medications

     i. Encourage ventilation of feelings about change in body image

     j. Monitor dysrhythmias

     k. Provide cooling blanket

     l. Monitor for infection

     m. Maintain a quiet environment

     n. Maintain seizure precautions

     o. Monitor for bleeding

     p. Protect from falls

     q. Encourage TCDB

     r. Allay anxiety

     s. Observe for uremic frost

     t. Provide skin and mouth care using plain water

     u. Monitor neurovital signs

8. Patient/family teaching goals; the patient will:

     a. Keep follow-up appointments

     b. Avoid use of over-the-counter medications

     c. Stop smoking

     d. Maintain ideal weight

     e. State the action, side effects, and scheduling of medications

     f. Recognize the signs and symptoms of renal failure, urinary tract infection, respiratory infection

     g. Avoid exposure to people with infections

     h. Alternate rest periods with activity

     i. Monitor self for infection

     j. Follow dietary recommendations and restrictions

     k. Maintain a quiet environemnt

     l. Seek help from community agencies and resources

9. Possible medical complications

     a. Chronic renal failure

     b. Decubiti

     c. Contractures

     d. Atelectasis

     e. Gastrointestinal hemorrhage

     f. Convulsions

     g. Dysrhythmias

     h. Cardiac arrest

     i. Pericarditis

     j. Potassium intoxication

     k. Pulmonary edema

     l. Pulmonary infection

m. CHF
n. Hypertension
10. Possible surgical interventions: none

P. Chronic renal failure
1. Definition: progressive, irreversible destruction of kidneys, resulting in loss of renal function
2. Possible etiology
    a. Recurrent urinary tract infection
    b. Exacerbations of nephritis
    c. Urinary tract obstructions
    d. Diabetes mellitus
    e. Hypertension
    f. Congenital abnormalities
    g. Systemic lupus erythematosus
    h. Nephrotoxins
    i. Dehydration
3. Pathophysiology
    a. Scarred nephrons are unable to absorb and secrete water, glucose, amino acids, ammonia, bicarbonate, and electrolytes
    b. First stage: renal reserve is diminished, but metabolic wastes do not accumulate although renal damage exists
    c. Second stage: renal insufficiency occurs and metabolic wastes begin to accumulate; kidneys are less able to correct metabolic imbalances
    d. Third stage: Uremia occurs, with decreased urine output, increased accumulation of metabolic wastes, and disturbed fluid, electrolyte, and acid-base balance
4. Possible clinical manifestations
    a. Muscle twitching
    b. Paresthesia
    c. Bone pain
    d. Pruritus
    e. Decreased urinary output
    f. Stomatitis
    g. Lethargy
    h. Convulsions
    i. Brittle nails and hair
    j. Kussmaul respirations
    k. Uremic frost
    l. Ecchymosis
5. Possible diagnostic test findings
    a. Urine chemistry: proteinuria, increased WBC, sodium; decreased and fixed specific gravity
    b. Blood chemistry: increased BUN, Cr, phosphorus, lipids; decreased calcium, CO_2, albumin
    c. ABGs: metabolic acidosis

    d. Hematology: decreased Hgb, Hct, platelets

    e. Glucose tolerance test: decreased

6. Medical management

    a. Diet therapy: low-protein, low-sodium, low-potassium, low-phosphorus, with high-calorie and high-carbohydrate; restricted fluids

    b. I.V. therapy: heparin lock

    c. Activity: as tolerated

    d. Monitoring: VS, UO, I/O

    e. Laboratory studies: BUN, Cr, potassium, sodium, Hgb, Hct, glucose, albumin, platelets

    f. Treatments: tepid baths

    g. Transfusion therapy: platelets

    h. Antibiotics: cefazolin (Ancef), cefoxitin (Mefoxin)

    i. Analgesics: oxycodone hydrochloride (Tylox)

    j. Diuretics: furosemide (Lasix)

    k. Antacids: aluminum hydroxide gel (Alternagel), magnesium and aluminum hydroxide (Maalox)

    l. Antiemetics: prochlorperazine (Compazine)

    m. Cation exchange resins: sodium polystyrene sulfonate (Kayexalate)

    n. Chelating agents: dimercaprol (BAL)

    o. Beta adrenergics: dopamine hydrochloride (Intropin)

    p. Anticonvulsants: phenytoin sodium (Dilantin)

    q. Peritoneal dialysis and hemodialysis

    r. Antipyretics: acetaminophen (Tylenol)

    s. Precautions: seizure

    t. Alkalinizing agent: sodium bicarbonate

    u. Cardioglycoside: digoxin (Lanoxin)

    v. Stool softeners: docusate sodium (Colace)

    w. Antiarrhythmics: procainamide (Pronestyl)

    x. Hematinic: ferrous sulfate (Feosol), iron dextran (Imferon), iron sorbitex (Jectofer)

    y. Vitamins: pyridoxine hydrochloride (vitamin B_6), ascorbic acid (vitamin C)

    z. Calcium supplements: calcium carbonate (Os-Cal)

7. Medical nursing interventions/responsibilities

    a. Maintain diet

    b. Restrict fluids

    c. Assess renal, respiratory, and cardiovascular status and fluid balance

    d. Monitor and record VS, UO, I/O, EKG, specific gravity, daily weight, laboratory studies, urine, stool, and emesis for occult blood, neurovital signs, neurovascular checks, urine for glucose and ketones

    e. Administer medications

    f. Encourage ventilation of feelings about chronicity of illness

    g. Provide treatments: tepid baths

    h. Maintain a cool and quiet environment

    i. Provide skin and mouth care using plain water

j. Maintain seizure precautions
k. Monitor for ecchymosis
l. Monitor for infection
m. Avoid intramuscular injections
n. Protect from falls

8. Patient/family teaching goals; the patient will:
a. Keep follow-up appointments
b. Stop smoking
c. Maintain ideal weight
d. State the action, side effects, and scheduling of medications
e. Recognize the signs and symptoms of infection
f. Avoid exposure to people with infection
g. Alternate rest periods with activity
h. Monitor self for infection
i. Follow dietary recommendations and restrictions
j. Promote a safe environment
k. Maintain a quiet environment
l. Seek help from community agencies and resources
m. Complete daily skin and mouth care

9. Possible medical complications
a. Dysrhythmias
b. Gastrointestinal bleeding
c. CHF
d. Pericardial effusion
e. Hyperphosphatemia
f. Pleural effusion
g. Dehydration
h. Hyperparathyroidism
i. Renal osteodystrophy
j. Uremia

10. Possible surgical interventions: kidney transplant (see page 199)

Q. Bladder cancer

1. Definition: malignant tumor that ulcerates mucosal lining of the bladder
2. Possible etiology
a. Exposure to industrial chemicals
b. Cigarette smoking
c. Chronic bladder irritation
d. Radiation
e. Excessive intake of coffee, phenacetin, sodium, saccharin, sodium cyclamate
f. Drug induced: cyclophosphamide (Cytoxan)
3. Pathophysiology
a. Unregulated cell growth and uncontrolled cell division in bladder's transitional epithelium around trigone result in the development of a neoplasm

  b. Tumor metastasizes to ureters, prostate gland, vagina, rectum, and periaortic lymph nodes

4. Possible clinical manifestations
  a. Painless hematuria
  b. Dysuria
  c. Frequency of urination
  d. Anuria
  e. Urgency of urination
  f. Chills
  g. Flank or pelvic pain
  h. Elevated temperature
  i. Peripheral edema

5. Possible diagnostic test findings
  a. Cystoscopy: presence of mass
  b. IVP: presence of mass or obstruction
  c. KUB: presence of mass or obstruction
  d. Cytologic exam: cytology positive for malignant cells
  e. Urine chemistry: hematuria
  f. Hematology: decreased RBCs, Hgb, Hct

6. Medical management
  a. I.V. therapy: heparin lock
  b. Activity: as tolerated
  c. Monitoring: VS, UO, I/O
  d. Laboratory studies: Hgb, Hct
  e. Radiation therapy
  f. Chemotherapy
  g. Treatments: Foley catheter
  h. Transfusion therapy: PRBC
  i. Sedatives: phenobarbital (Luminal)
  j. Antispasmotics: phenazopyridine (Pyridium)
  k. Antineoplastics: 5-fluorouracil (5FU), methotrexate (MTX), bleomycin (Blenoxane), thiotepa (TSPA), doxorubicin hydrochloride (Adriamycin)

7. Medical nursing interventions/responsibilities
  a. Maintain diet
  b. Force fluids
  c. Administer I.V. fluids
  d. Assess renal status
  e. Monitor and record VS, UO, I/O, laboratory studies
  f. Administer medications
  g. Encourage ventilation of feelings about fear of dying
  h. Provide postchemotherapeutic and/or postradiation nursing care: provide skin, mouth, and perineal care; encourage dietary intake; administer antiemetics and antidiarrheals; monitor for bleeding, infection, and electrolyte imbalance; provide rest periods

8. Patient/family teaching goals; the patient will:
    a. Keep follow-up appointments
    b. Stop smoking
    c. Maintain ideal weight
    d. State the action, side effects, and scheduling of medications
    e. Recognize the signs and symptoms of urinary tract infection and renal failure
    f. Avoid exposure to people with infections
    g. Alternate rest periods with activity
    h. Monitor self for infection
    i. Follow dietary recommendations and restrictions
    j. Seek help from community agencies and resources
9. Possible medical complications
    a. Ureteral obstruction
    b. Vesicorectal and vesicovaginal fistulas
10. Possible surgical interventions
    a. Ureterosigmoidostomy (see page 203)
    b. Ileal conduit (see page 204)
    c. Cutaneous ureterostomy (see page 204)
    d. Cystectomy

R. Benign prostatic hypertrophy (BPH)

1. Definition: hyperplasia of lateral and subcervical lobes of the prostate gland that results in enlargement of the structure
2. Possible etiology
    a. Unknown
    b. Hormonal
3. Pathophysiology
    a. Enlarged prostate gland compresses urethra, resulting in urinary obstruction and retention
    b. Obstruction causes hydroureter and hydronephrosis
4. Possible clinical manifestations
    a. Nocturia
    b. Urgency, frequency, and burning on urination
    c. Decreased force and amount of stream
    d. Hesitancy
    e. Dysuria
    f. Urinary retention
    g. Urinary tract infection
    h. Dribbling
5. Possible diagnostic test findings
    a. Rectal examination: enlarged prostate gland by palpation
    b. Urine chemistry: presence of bacteria, hematuria, alkaline pH, increased specific gravity
    c. Blood chemistry: increased BUN, Cr
    d. PSP: decreased

    e. IVP: urethral obstruction, hydronephrosis

    f. Cystoscopy: enlarged prostate gland, obstructed urine flow, urine stasis

6. Medical management

    a. Diet therapy: force fluids

    b. Position: semi-Fowler

    c. Activity: as tolerated

    d. Monitoring: VS, UO, I/O

    e. Laboratory studies: BUN, Cr

    f. Treatments: Foley catheter, hot baths

    g. Antibiotics: trimethoprim and sulfamethoxazole (Bactrim), cephalexin (Keflex)

    h. Analgesics: oxycodone hydrochloride (Tylox)

    i. Urinary antiseptics: phenazopyridine (Pyridium)

    j. Antianxiety: diazepam (Valium)

7. Medical nursing interventions/responsibilities

    a. Force fluids

    b. Assess fluid balance

    c. Maintain semi-Fowler position

    d. Monitor and record: VS, UO, I/O, laboratory studies

    e. Administer medications

    f. Encourage ventilation of feelings about change in body image and fear of sexual dysfunction

    g. Maintain position and patency of Foley catheter to straight drainage

    h. Maintain activity as tolerated

    i. Provide hot baths

    j. Provide privacy while urinating

    k. Monitor for urinary tract infection

8. Patient/family teaching goals; the patient will:

    a. Keep follow-up appointments

    b. Stop smoking

    c. Maintain ideal weight

    d. State the action, side effects, and scheduling of medications

    e. Recognize the signs and symptoms of urinary retention and infection

9. Possible medical complications

    a. Chronic renal failure

    b. Hydronephrosis

    c. Hydroureter

    d. Renal calculi

    e. Cystitis

10. Possible surgical interventions

    a. Suprapubic cystotomy with insertion of suprapubic catheter (see page 202)

    b. Transurethral resection of prostate gland (TURP) (see page 202)

    c. Prostatectomy (see page 202)

Points to Remember

Renal disease alters fluid balance.

Sodium and potassium balance are always affected in renal system disorders.

Renal system disease can alter the renin-angiotensin system, which controls blood pressure.

Illnesses that alter fluid balance affect kidney function.

Specific gravity, daily weight, and accurate output are independent, objective nursing assessments for renal function.

Glossary

Anuria — absence of urine output.

Hematuria — presence of blood in urine.

Oliguria — urine output of less than 30 ml/hour.

Pyuria — presence of pus in the urine.

Renal colic — flank pain that radiates to the groin.

Respiratory System

Learning Objectives

After studying this section, the reader should be able to:

• Describe the psychosocial impact of respiratory system disorders.

• Differentiate between modifiable and nonmodifiable risk factors in the development of a respiratory system disorder.

• List three potential and three actual nursing diagnoses for the patient with a respiratory system disorder.

• Identify the medical and surgical nursing interventions/ responsibilities for the patient with a respiratory system disorder.

• Write three teaching goals for the patient with a respiratory system disorder.

VII. Respiratory System

A. Anatomy and physiology

1. Nose
   a. Filters out particles
   b. Humidifies inspired air
   c. Contains olfactory receptor site
2. Paranasal sinuses
   a. Air-filled, cilia-lined cavities
   b. Function: to trap particles
3. Pharynx
   a. Serves as passageway to digestive and respiratory tracts
   b. Maintains air pressure in middle ear
   c. Contains mucosal lining that humidifies and warms inspired air and traps particles
4. Larynx
   a. Known as "voice box;" connects upper and lower airways
   b. Contains vocal cords of larynx that produce sounds and initiate the cough reflex
5. Trachea
   a. Consists of smooth muscle; contains C-shaped cartilagenous rings
   b. Connects larynx to bronchi
6. Bronchi and bronchioles
   a. They are formed by branching of trachea
   b. Right main bronchus is slightly larger and more vertical than left
   c. Bronchioles branch into terminal bronchioles, which end in alveoli
7. Alveoli
   a. Clustered microscopic sacs enveloped by capillaries
   b. Site for exchange of gases
   c. Coating of surfactant reduces surface tension to keep alveoli from collapsing
   d. Diffusion of gases occurs across alveolar-capillary membrane
8. Lungs
   a. They are composed of three lobes on right side and two lobes on left side
   b. They are covered by pleura
   c. The concentration gradient regulates air exchange
9. Pleura
   a. Visceral pleura covers the lungs
   b. Parietal pleura lines the thoracic cavity
   c. Pleural fluid lubricates the pleura to reduce friction during respiration

B. Physical assessment findings

1. Subjective data that often accompany respiratory disorders
   a. Difficulty breathing
   b. Chest pain

      c. Voice change
      d. Dysphagia
      e. Fatigue
      f. Change in weight
      g. Cough
  2. Objective data to evaluate in respiratory disorders
      a. Dyspnea
      b. Sputum
      c. Clubbing of fingers
      d. Adventitious sounds: rales, rhonchi, wheezing, and pleural friction rub
      e. Fremitus
      f. Crepitus
      g. Pattern and character of respirations
      h. Thoracic anatomy
      i. Change in mentation
      j. Skin color and temperature

C. Diagnostic tests and procedures used to evaluate respiratory disorders
  1. Bronchoscopy
      a. Definition/purpose: direct visualization of the trachea and bronchial tree using a bronchoscope
      b. Nursing interventions/responsibilities: before procedure, withhold food and fluids; allay anxiety; after procedure, assess cough and gag reflex; assess sputum; assess respiratory status; withhold food and fluids until gag reflex returns; assess vasovagal response
  2. Chest X-ray (CXR)
      a. Definition/purpose: radiographic picture of lung tissue
      b. Nursing interventions/responsibilities: assess patient's ability to inhale and hold breath; remove jewelry
  3. Pulmonary angiography
      a. Definition/purpose: radiographic examination of the pulmonary circulation after injection of radiopaque dye through a catheter
      b. Nursing interventions/responsibilities: before procedure, assess allergies to radiopaque dyes, iodine, and seafood; instruct patient he may feel flushing in the face or burning in the throat after dye is injected; after procedure, assess peripheral neurovascular status; monitor injection site for bleeding
  4. Sputum studies
      a. Definition/purpose: microscopic evaluation of sputum that includes culture and sensitivity, gram stain, and acid-fast bacillus
      b. Nursing interventions/responsibilities: obtain early-morning sterile specimen from suctioning or expectoration
  5. Thoracentesis
      a. Definition/purpose: needle aspiration of intrapleural fluid under local anesthesia for purposes of specimen examination or removal of pleural fluid

    b. Nursing interventions/responsibilities: during procedure, reassure patient and maintain proper position of patient; after procedure, assess respiratory status

6. Pulmonary function tests (PFTs)
    a. Definition/purpose: measure of lung volumes, ventilation, and diffusing capacity
    b. Nursing interventions/responsibilities: document bronchodilators or narcotics used before testing; allay anxiety during testing

7. Arterial blood gases (ABGs)
    a. Definition/purpose: assessment of arterial blood for tissue oxygenation, ventilation, and acid-base status
    b. Nursing interventions/responsibilities: document temperature, oxygen, and assisted mechanical ventilation used before testing; after procedure apply pressure to site for 5 minutes; apply pressure dressing

8. Lung scan
    a. Definition/purpose: visual imaging of distribution of blood flow in the lungs after inhalation or I.V. injection of radioisotopes
    b. Nursing interventions/responsibilities: before procedure, allay anxiety; assess patient's ability to lie still during procedure; after procedure, inspect catheter insertion site for bleeding

9. Mantoux intradermal skin test
    a. Definition/purpose: administration of tuberculin to detect the presence of tuberculosis antibodies
    b. Nursing interventions/responsibilities: document current dermatitis or rashes; document history of positive results in past skin testing; circle and record test site; document date for follow-up reading

10. Laryngoscopy
    a. Definition/purpose: direct visualization of the larynx using a laryngoscope
    b. Nursing interventions/responsibilities: before procedure, withhold food or fluids; after procedure, assess respiratory status; allay anxiety

11. Lung biopsy
    a. Definition/purpose: percutaneous removal of a small amount of lung tissue for histologic evaluation
    b. Nursing interventions/responsibilities: before procedure, withhold food and fluids; obtain written, informed consent; after procedure, observe patient for signs of pneumothorax and air embolism; assess patient for hemoptysis and hemorrhage; monitor vital signs (VS); assess site for bleeding

12. Hematologic studies
    a. Definition/purpose: laboratory analysis of blood sample for red blood cells (RBC), white blood cells (WBC), prothrombin time (PT), partial thromboplastin time (PTT), erythrocyte sedimentation rate (ESR), platelets, hemoglobin (Hgb), hematocrit (Hct)
    b. Nursing interventions/responsibilities: assess site for bleeding; note current drug therapy

13. Blood chemistry
   a. Definition/purpose: laboratory analysis of blood sample for potassium, sodium, calcium, phosphorus, glucose, bicarbonate, blood urea nitrogen (BUN), creatinine (Cr), protein, albumin, and osmolality
   b. Nursing interventions/responsibilities: before procedure, withhold food and fluids as ordered; after procedure, monitor site for bleeding

D. Possible psychosocial impact of respiratory disorders
   1. Developmental impact
      a. Decreased self-esteem
      b. Fear of dying
   2. Economic impact
      a. Disruption or loss of employment
      b. Cost of hospitalizations and home health care
   3. Occupational and recreational impact
      a. Restrictions in work activity
      b. Change in leisure activities
   4. Social impact
      a. Change in sexual function
      b. Social isolation
      c. Change in role performance

E. Possible risk factors
   1. Modifiable risk factors
      a. Crowded living conditions
      b. Inadequate knowledge of risk factors
      c. Exposure to chemical and environmental pollutants
      d. Cigarette or pipe smoking
      e. Use of chewing tobacco
      f. Alcohol abuse
   2. Nonmodifiable risk factors
      a. Aging process
      b. History of allergies
      c. History of previous respiratory illness
      d. Family history of respiratory illness
      e. Family history of allergies

F. Possible nursing diagnoses for the patient with respiratory disorders
   1. Actual nursing diagnoses
      a. Impaired physical mobility
      b. Alteration in tissue perfusion: cerebral
      c. Alteration in tissue perfusion: peripheral
      d. Alteration in tissue perfusion: cardiopulmonary
      e. Sleep pattern disturbance

2. Potential nursing diagnoses
   a. Ineffective breathing patterns
   b. Impaired gas exchange
   c. Ineffective airway clearance
   d. Anxiety
   e. Fear
   f. Activity intolerance
   g. Impaired verbal communication
   h. Noncompliance

G. Surgical intervention: laryngectomy
1. Definition
   a. Partial laryngectomy: surgical excision of a lesion on one vocal cord
   b. Total laryngectomy: surgical removal of the larynx, hyoid bone, and tracheal rings with closure of the pharynx and formation of a permanent tracheostomy
2. Preoperative surgical nursing interventions/responsibilities
   a. Complete patient and family preoperative teaching: assess understanding of surgical procedure; explain operating room (OR), recovery room (RR), preoperative and postoperative routine; demonstrate postoperative turning, coughing, and deep breathing (TCDB), splinting, leg exercises, and range-of-motion (ROM) exercises; explain postoperative need for drainage tubes, surgical dressings, oxygen therapy, I.V. therapy, and pain control
   b. Complete preoperative check list
   c. Administer preoperative medications
   d. Allay patient and family anxiety about surgery
   e. Document patient history and physical assessment data base
   f. Establish methods of communication: writing, call bell
   g. Encourage ventilation of feelings about change in body image, loss of voice
3. Postoperative surgical nursing interventions/responsibilities
   a. Assess respiratory status
   b. Assess pain and administer postoperative analgesic
   c. Progress diet as tolerated: increased calories and protein
   d. Administer I.V. fluids and nasogastric (NG) tube feedings
   e. Allay anxiety
   f. Assess surgical dressing and change as directed
   g. Reinforce TCDB
   h. Maintain semi-Fowler position
   i. Assess for return of peristalsis
   j. Provide pulmonary toilet: tracheal suction
   k. Progress activity as tolerated
   l. Administer oxygen via high humidity tracheostomy mask
   m. Monitor VS, urinary output (UO), intake and output (I/O), laboratory studies

     n. Monitor and maintain position and patency of drainage tubes: wound drainage
     o. Assess color, amount, consistency of sputum
     p. Encourage ventilation of feelings about change in body image and loss of voice
     q. Provide oral hygiene
     r. Reinforce method of communication established preoperatively
     s. Reinforce speech therapy
     t. Assess gag and cough reflex and ability to swallow
     u. Provide stoma and laryngectomy care
     v. Reinforce increased intake of fluids
     w. Assess for hemorrhage and edema in neck

4. Possible surgical complications
     a. Hemorrhage
     b. Atelectasis
     c. Pneumonia
     d. Aspiration

5. Patient/family postoperative teaching goals; the patient will:
     a. Keep follow-up appointments
     b. Communicate using esophageal speech or artificial larynx
     c. State the action, side effects, and scheduling of medications
     d. Recognize the signs and symptoms of infection
     e. Avoid swimming, showering, and use of aerosal sprays
     f. Complete daily stoma and laryngectomy care
     g. Suction laryngectomy using clean technique
     h. Protect the neck from injury
     i. Demonstrate ways to prevent debris from entering the stoma
     j. Seek help from community agencies and resources

H. Surgical intervention: radical neck dissection

1. Definition: surgical excision of the sternocleidomastoid and omohyoid muscles, muscles of the floor of the mouth, submaxillary gland, internal jugular vein, external carotid artery, cervical chain of lymph nodes in addition to laryngectomy
2. Preoperative surgical nursing interventions/responsibilities
     a. Complete patient and family preoperative teaching: assess understanding of surgical procedure; explain OR, RR, preoperative and postoperative routine; demonstrate postoperative TCDB, splinting, leg exercises, and ROM; explain postoperative need for drainage tubes, surgical dressings, oxygen therapy, I.V. therapy, and pain control
     b. Complete preoperative check list
     c. Administer preoperative medications
     d. Allay patient and family anxiety about surgery
     e. Document patient history and physical assessment data base
     f. Establish method of communication: writing, call bell

3. Postoperative surgical nursing interventions/responsibilities
   a. Assess cardiac, respiratory, and neurologic status
   b. Assess pain and administer postoperative analgesic
   c. Progress diet as tolerated
   d. Administer I.V. fluids, NG tube feedings, and transfusion therapy
   e. Allay anxiety
   f. Assess surgical dressing and change as directed
   g. Reinforce TCDB
   h. Maintain high-Fowler position
   i. Assess for return of peristalsis
   j. Provide pulmonary toilet: tracheal suction
   k. Maintain activity: as tolerated, active and passive ROM, isometric exercises
   l. Administer oxygen via high humidity tracheostomy mask
   m. Monitor VS, UO, I/O, laboratory studies
   n. Monitor and maintain position and patency of drainage tubes: NG, Foley, wound drainage
   o. Assess gag and cough reflex and ability to swallow
   p. Encourage ventilation of feelings about change in body image, loss of voice
   q. Provide stoma and laryngectomy care
   r. Reinforce increased intake of fluids
   s. Assess for hemorrhage and edema in neck
   t. Provide suture line care
   u. Reinforce method of communication established preoperatively
   v. Reinforce speech therapy
4. Possible surgical complications
   a. Tracheostomy stenosis
   b. Aspiration
   c. Pneumonia
   d. Hemorrhage
5. Postoperative teaching goals; the patient will:
   a. Keep follow-up appointments
   b. Communicate using esophageal speech or artificial larynx
   c. State the action, side effects, and scheduling of medications
   d. Recognize the signs and symptoms of infection and tracheostomy stenosis
   e. Avoid showers, swimming, and use of aerosol sprays
   f. Protect neck from injury
   g. Seek help from community agencies and resources
   h. Suction laryngectomy using clean technique
   i. Complete daily incision, stoma, and laryngectomy care
   j. Demonstrate ways to prevent debris from entering the stoma
   k. Complete daily ROM exercises for arms, shoulders, and neck
   l. Use specialized appliances: artificial larynx

I. Surgical intervention: pulmonary resections
1. Definition
    a. Lobectomy: surgical removal of one lobe of the lung
    b. Wedge resection: surgical removal of a wedge-shaped section of a lobe
    c. Pneumonectomy: surgical removal of a lung
2. Preoperative surgical nursing interventions/responsibilities
    a. Complete patient and family preoperative teaching: assess understanding of surgical procedure; explain OR, RR, preoperative and postoperative routine; demonstrate postoperative TCDB, splinting, leg exercises, and ROM; explain postoperative need for drainage tubes, chest tubes, surgical dressings, oxygen therapy, I.V. therapy, and pain control
    b. Complete preoperative check list
    c. Administer preoperative medications
    d. Allay patient and family anxiety about surgery
    e. Document patient history and physical assessment data base
3. Postoperative surgical nursing interventions/responsibilities
    a. Assess cardiac and respiratory status
    b. Assess pain and administer postoperative analgesic
    c. Progress diet as tolerated
    d. Administer I.V. fluids
    e. Allay anxiety
    f. Assess surgical dressing and change as directed
    g. Reinforce TCDB and splinting of incision
    h. Maintain position: on back or operative side for pneumonectomy patient; on back or unoperative side for lobectomy or wedge resection patient
    i. Assess for return of peristalsis
    j. Provide pulmonary toilet: incentive spirometry, suction, chest physiotherapy (CPT), postural drainage
    k. Maintain activity: as tolerated, active and passive ROM, isometric exercises
    l. Administer oxygen and maintain endotracheal tube to ventilator
    m. Monitor and record VS, UO, I/O, laboratory studies, EKG, hemodynamic variables
    n. Monitor and maintain position and patency of drainage tubes: NG, Foley, chest tube
    o. Assess chest tube insertion site for subcutaneous air, drainage
    p. Encourage ventilation of feelings about fear of dying
    q. Administer antibiotics
4. Possible surgical complications
    a. Hemorrhage
    b. Pneumonia
5. Patient/family postoperative teaching goals; the patient will:
    a. Keep follow-up appointments
    b. Maintain regular exercise program

    c. Stop smoking
    d. Maintain ideal weight
    e. State the action, side effects, and scheduling of medications
    f. Recognize the signs and symptoms of infection and respiratory distress
    g. Complete daily incision care
    h. Maintain active ROM to operative shoulder

J. Surgical intervention: embolectomy
    1. Definition: removal of an embolus from an artery using a balloon-tipped catheter (Fogarty)
    2. Preoperative surgical nursing interventions/responsibilities
       a. Complete patient and family preoperative teaching: assess understanding of surgical procedure; explain OR, RR, preoperative and postoperative routine; demonstrate postoperative TCDB, splinting, leg exercises, and ROM; explain postoperative need for drainage tubes, surgical dressings, oxygen therapy, I.V. therapy, and pain control
       b. Complete preoperative check list
       c. Administer preoperative medications
       d. Allay patient and family anxiety about surgery
       e. Document patient history and physical assessment data base
       f. Obtain baseline vascular assessment
       g. Administer anticoagulants
       h. Administer antispasmodics
       i. Administer thrombolytics
       j. Provide bed cradle
       k. Avoid bumping the bed
       l. Maintain extremity in slightly dependent position
    3. Postoperative surgical nursing interventions/responsibilities
       a. Assess cardiac, respiratory, and neurologic status
       b. Assess pain and administer postoperative analgesic
       c. Progress diet as tolerated
       d. Administer I.V. fluids
       e. Allay anxiety
       f. Assess surgical dressing and change as directed
       g. Reinforce TCDB
       h. Maintain semi-Fowler position
       i. Assess for return of peristalsis
       j. Provide pulmonary toilet: incentive spirometry
       k. Maintain activity: as tolerated, active and passive ROM, isometric exercises
       l. Administer oxygen
       m. Monitor and record VS, UO, I/O, laboratory studies, neurovascular checks
       n. Administer anticoagulants
       o. Provide bed cradle

     p. Assess site for bleeding
     q. Maintain pressure dressing
  4. Possible surgical complications
     a. Hemorrhage
     b. Embolus
     c. Thrombus
  5. Patient/family postoperative teaching goals; the patient will:
     a. Keep follow-up appointments
     b. Maintain regular exercise program
     c. Stop smoking
     d. Maintain ideal weight
     e. State the action, side effects, and scheduling of medications
     f. Recognize the signs and symptoms of infection and bleeding
     g. Avoid prolonged periods of sitting
     h. State cautions of long-term anticoagulant therapy
     i. Complete daily incision care

K. Surgical intervention: vena caval filter/plication of inferior vena cava
  1. Definition
     a. Vena caval filter: surgical insertion of an intracaval filter (umbrella) to partially occlude the inferior vena cava and prevent pulmonary emboli
     b. Plication: surgical suturing and placement of Teflon clips to partially occlude the inferior vena cava and to strain the blood to prevent pulmonary emboli
  2. Preoperative surgical nursing interventions/responsibilities
     a. Complete patient and family preoperative teaching: assess understanding of surgical procedure; explain OR, RR, preoperative and postoperative routine; demonstrate postoperative TCDB, splinting, leg exercises, and ROM; explain postoperative need for drainage tubes, surgical dressings, oxygen therapy, I.V. therapy, and pain control
     b. Complete preoperative check list
     c. Administer preoperative medications
     d. Allay patient and family anxiety about surgery
     e. Document patient history and physical assessment data base
  3. Postoperative surgical nursing interventions/responsibilities
     a. Assess cardiac and respiratory status
     b. Assess pain and administer postoperative analgesic
     c. Progress diet as tolerated
     d. Administer I.V. fluids
     e. Allay anxiety
     f. Assess surgical dressing and change as directed
     g. Reinforce TCDB
     h. Maintain semi-Fowler position, with foot of bed elevated
     i. Assess for return of peristalsis
     j. Provide pulmonary toilet: incentive spirometry

   k. Maintain activity: as tolerated, active and passive ROM, isometric
       exercises
   l. Administer oxygen
   m. Monitor and record VS, UO, I/O, laboratory studies, neurovascular
       checks
   n. Assess insertion site for bleeding and hematoma
   o. Assess peripheral edema
   p. Apply antiembolitic stockings
   q. Avoid hip flexion
4. Possible surgical complications
   a. Embolism
   b. Infection
5. Patient/family postoperative teaching goals; the patient will:
   a. Keep follow-up appointments
   b. Stop smoking
   c. Maintain ideal weight
   d. State the action, side effects, and scheduling of medications
   e. Recognize the signs and symptoms of infection and edema
   f. Avoid sitting for prolonged periods or crossing legs when sitting
   g. Complete daily incision care
   h. Ambulate daily
   i. Elevate legs when sitting
   j. Wear antiembolitic stockings
   k. Adhere to long-term anticoagulant therapy

L. Pneumonia
1. Definition: bacterial, viral, or fungal infection that causes inflammation of
    the alveolar spaces
2. Possible etiology
   a. Organisms: *E. coli, H. influenzae, S. aureus*
   b. Aspiration of food
   c. Aspiration of fluid
   d. Chemical irritants
3. Pathophysiology
   a. Microorganisms enter the alveolar spaces by droplet inhalation
   b. Inflammation occurs and alveolar fluid increases
   c. Ventilation decreases as secretions thicken
4. Possible clinical manifestations
   a. Cough
   b. Malaise
   c. Chills
   d. Shortness of breath
   e. Dyspnea
   f. Elevated temperature
   g. Rales
   h. Rhonchi

    i. Pleural friction rub

    j. Pleuritic pain

    k. Sputum production: rusty, green, or bloody (pneumococcal pneumonia); yellow-green (bronchopneumonia)

5. Possible diagnostic test findings

    a. Sputum studies: identification of organism

    b. CXR: pulmonary infiltrates

    c. Hematology: increased WBC, ESR

    d. ABGs: hypoxemia, respiratory alkalosis

6. Medical management

    a. Diet therapy: high-calorie, high-protein; force fluids

    b. I.V. therapy: hydration, heparin lock

    c. Oxygen therapy

    d. Intubation and mechanical ventilation

    e. Position: semi-Fowler

    f. Activity: bed rest, active and passive ROM, isometric exercises

    g. Monitoring: VS, UO, I/O

    h. Laboratory studies: WBC, sputum culture, blood culture, throat culture

    i. Nutritional support: I.V. hyperalimentation (IVH)

    j. Treatments: Foley catheter, CPT, postural drainage, incentive spirometry

    k. Antibiotics: pencillin G potassium (Pentids), ampicillin (Omnipen)

    l. Antipyretics: aspirin (Ecotrin), acetaminophen (Tylenol)

7. Medical nursing interventions/responsibilities

    a. Maintain diet

    b. Force fluids to 3 to 4 liters/day

    c. Administer I.V. fluids

    d. Administer oxygen

    e. Provide pulmonary toilet: suction, TCDB

    f. Assess respiratory status

    g. Maintain semi-Fowler position

    h. Monitor and record VS, UO, I/O, laboratory studies

    i. Administer medications

    j. Encourage ventilation of feelings about fear of suffocation

    n. Monitor color, consistency, and amount of sputum

    o. Allay anxiety

    p. Prevent spread of infection

    q. Provide oral hygiene

8. Patient/family teaching goals; the patient will:

    a. Keep follow-up appointments

    b. Stop smoking

    c. State the action, side effects, and scheduling of medications

    d. Recognize the signs and symptoms of respiratory infections

    e. Avoid exposure to people with infections

    f. Alternate rest periods with activity

    g. Monitor self for infection

     h. Follow dietary recommendations and restrictions
     i. Increase fluid intake to 3,000 ml/day
  9. Possible medical complications
     a. Congestive heart failure (CHF)
     b. Pulmonary edema
     c. Respiratory failure
10. Possible surgical interventions: none

M. Chronic obstructive pulmonary disease (COPD)

  1. Definition
     a. COPD is group of diseases that result in persistent obstruction of bronchial air flow
     b. They include emphysema, asthma, bronchiectasis, and bronchitis
     c. Stimulant to breathe is low PO_2 instead of increased PCO_2
  2. Possible etiology
     a. Congential weakness
     b. Respiratory irritants: smoke, polluted air, chemical irritants
     c. Respiratory tract infections
     d. Genetic predisposition
  3. Pathophysiology
     a. Bronchiectasis: infection destroys the bronchial mucosa, which is replaced by fibrous scar tissue; loss of resilience and dilation of airways causes pooling of secretions, obstruction of air flow, and decreased perfusion
     b. Asthma: irritants to bronchial tree cause bronchoconstriction, resulting in narrowed inflamed airways, dyspnea, and mucus production
     c. Bronchitis: excessive bronchial mucus production causes chronic or recurrent productive cough
     d. Emphysema: destruction of elastin alters alveolar walls and narrows airways, resulting in enlargement of air spaces distal to terminal bronchioles, trapped air, and coalesced alveoli
  4. Possible clinical manifestations
     a. Cough
     b. Dyspnea
     c. Sputum production
     d. Weight loss
     e. Barrel chest (emphysema)
     f. Hemoptysis
     g. Exertional dyspnea
     h. Clubbing of fingers
     i. Malaise
     j. Wheezes
     k. Rales
     l. Anemia
     m. Anxiety
     n. Diaphoresis

     o. Use of accessory muscles
     p. Orthopnea
5. Possible diagnostic test findings
     a. CXR: congestion, hyperinflation
     b. ABGs: respiratory acidosis, hypoxemia
     c. Sputum studies: positive identification of organism
     d. PFTs: increased residual volume, increased functional residual capacity, decreased vital capacity
6. Medical management
     a. Diet therapy: high-protein, high-carbohydrate, high-vitamin C; force fluids to 3,000 ml/day
     b. I.V. therapy: heparin lock
     c. Oxygen therapy: 2 to 3 liters/minute
     d. Intubation and mechanical ventilation
     e. Position: high-Fowler
     f. Activity: as tolerated
     g. Monitoring: VS, UO, I/O
     h. Laboratory studies: ABGs, WBC, sputum studies
     i. Treatments: CPT, postural drainage, intermittent positive pressure breathing (IPPB), incentive spirometry
     j. Antibiotics: ampicillin (Omnipen), tetracycline (Achromycin)
     k. Antacids: aluminum hydroxide gel (Alternagel)
     l. Bronchodilators: terbutaline (Brethine), aminophylline (Aminodur), isoproterenol (Isuprel)
     m. Steroids: hydrocortisone (Solu-Cortef), methylprednisolone (Solu-Medrol)
     n. Expectorants: guaifenesin (Robitussin)
     o. Beta-adrenergic drugs: epinephrine (Adrenalin)
7. Medical nursing interventions/responsibilities
     a. Maintain diet
     b. Force fluids
     c. Administer low-flow oxygen
     d. Provide pulmonary toilet: CPT, IPPB, TCDB, postural drainage, incentive spirometry, suction
     e. Assess respiratory status
     f. Reinforce pursed-lip breathing
     g. Maintain high-Fowler position
     h. Monitor and record VS, UO, I/O, laboratory studies
     j. Administer medications
     k. Encourage ventilation of feelings about fear of suffocation
     l. Activity as tolerated
     m. Assess color, amount, and consistency of sputum
     n. Allay anxiety
     o. Weigh daily
8. Patient/family teaching goals; the patient will:
     a. Keep follow-up appointments
     b. Maintain regular exercise program

      c. Stop smoking
      d. Maintain ideal weight
      e. State the action, side effects, and scheduling of medications
      f. Identify and reduce stress
      g. Recognize the signs and symptoms of respiratory infection and hypoxia
      h. Adhere to activity limitations
      i. Avoid exposure to people with infections
      j. Alternate rest periods with activity
      k. Monitor self for infection
      l. Follow dietary recommendations and restrictions
      m. Maintain a quiet environment
      n. Seek help from community agencies and resources
      o. Demonstrate pursed-lip and diaphragmatic breathing
      p. Avoid exposure to chemical irritants and pollutants
      q. Demonstrate deep-breathing and coughing exercises
  9. Possible medical complications
      a. Emphysema: pulmonary hypertension, right-sided congestive heart failure, spontaneous pneumothorax
      b. Carbon dioxide narcosis
      c. Acute respiratory failure
      d. Pneumonia
10. Possible surgical interventions: none

N. Adult respiratory distress syndrome (ARDS, shock lung)
  1. Definition: clinical syndrome of respiratory insufficiency
  2. Possible etiology
      a. Viral pneumonia
      b. Fat emboli
      c. Sepsis
      d. Decreased surfactant production
      e. Fluid overload
      f. Shock
      g. Trauma
      h. Neurologic injuries
      i. Oxygen toxicity
  3. Pathophysiology
      a. Damaged capillary membranes cause interstitial edema and intra-alveolar hemorrhage
      b. Decreased gas exchange results
      c. Cellular damage causes decreased surfactant production, resulting in hypoxemia
  4. Possible clinical manifestations
      a. Dyspnea
      b. Tachypnea
      c. Cyanosis
      d. Cough

   e. Rales
   f. Rhonchi
   g. Anxiety
   h. Restlessness
   i. Decreased breath sounds
5. Possible diagnostic test findings
   a. ABGs: respiratory acidosis, hypoxemia that does not respond to increased percentage of oxygen
   b. CXR: interstitial edema
   c. Sputum studies: presence of organism
   d. Blood cultures: presence of organism
6. Medical management
   a. Diet therapy: restrict fluid intake
   b. I.V. therapy: heparin lock
   c. Oxygen therapy
   d. Intubation and mechanical ventilation using positive end expiratory pressure (PEEP)
   e. Position: high-Fowler
   f. Activity: bed rest, active ROM, isometric exercises
   g. Monitoring: VS, UO, I/O, CVP, EKG, hemodynamic variables
   h. Laboratory studies: ABGs, sputum studies, blood cultures, Hgb, Hct
   i. Nutritional support: IVH
   j. Treatments: Foley catheter, CPT, postural drainage, suction
   k. Transfusion therapy: platelets, packed red blood cells (PRBC)
   l. Antibiotics: amoxicillin (Amoxil), ampicillin (Omnipen)
   m. Analgesics: morphine sulfate
   n. Diuretics: furosemide (Lasix), ethacrynic acid (Edecrin)
   o. Anticoagulants: heparin (Lipo-Hepin)
   p. Steroids: hydrocortisone (Solu-Cortef), methylprednisolone (Solu-Medrol)
   q. Antacids: aluminum hydroxide gel (Alternagel)
7. Medical nursing interventions/responsibilities
   a. Maintain fluid restrictions
   b. Administer I.V. fluids
   c. Monitor mechanical ventilation
   d. Provide pulmonary toilet: suction, TCDB, postural drainage
   e. Assess respiratory status
   f. Maintain high-Fowler position
   g. Monitor and record VS, UO, CVP, hemodynamic variables, I/O, specific gravity, laboratory studies
   h. Administer IVH
   i. Administer medications
   j. Encourage ventilation of feelings about fear of suffocation
   k. Organize nursing care to allow rest periods
   l. Weigh daily

      m. Allay anxiety

      n. Maintain bed rest

  8. Patient/family teaching goals; the patient will:

      a. Keep follow-up appointments

      b. Stop smoking

      c. State the action, side effects, and scheduling of medications

      d. Recognize the signs and symptoms of respiratory distress

      e. Adhere to activity limitations

      f. Avoid exposure to people with respiratory infections

      g. Alternate rest periods with activity

      h. Monitor self for infection

      i. Demonstrate deep breathing and coughing exercises

      j. Avoid exposure to chemical irritants and pollutants

  9. Possible medical complications

      a. Pulmonary edema

      b. Atelectasis

  10. Possible surgical interventions: none

O. Tuberculosis (pulmonary)

  1. Definition: airborne, infectious, communicable disease that can occur acutely or chronically

  2. Possible etiology: *Mycobacterium tuberculosis*

  3. Pathophysiology

      a. Alveoli become the focus of infection from inhaled droplets containing bacteria

      b. Tubercle bacilli multiply, spread through the lymphatics, and drain into the systemic circulation

      c. In the lung tissue, macrophages surround the bacilli and form tubercles

      d. Tubercles go through the process of caseation, liquefaction, and cavitation

  4. Possible clinical manifestations

      a. Fatigue

      b. Malaise

      c. Irritability

      d. Night sweats

      e. Tachycardia

      f. Weight loss

      g. Anorexia

      h. Cough

      i. Yellow and mucoid sputum production

      j. Dyspnea

      k. Hemoptysis

      l. Rales

      m. Elevated temperature

5. Possible diagnostic test findings
    a. CXR: active or calcified lesions
    b. Sputum cultures: positive acid-fast bacillus; positive *M. tuberculosis*
    c. Hematology: increased WBC, ESR
    d. Mantoux skin test: positive
6. Medical management
    a. Diet therapy: high-carbohydrate, high-protein, high-vitamin B_6
    b. I.V. therapy: heparin lock
    c. Activity: bed rest, active ROM, isometric exercises
    d. Monitoring: VS, UO, I/O
    e. Laboratory studies: ABGs, sputum studies
    f. Treatments: CPT, postural drainage, incentive spirometry
    g. Precautions: respiratory
    h. Antibiotics: streptomycin
    i. Antituberculosis: isoniazid (INH), ethambutol (Myambutol), rifampin (Rifadin)
7. Medical nursing interventions/responsibilities
    a. Maintain diet
    b. Provide pulmonary toilet: suction, TCDB, CPT, postural drainage
    c. Assess respiratory status
    d. Monitor and record VS, UO, I/O, laboratory studies
    e. Administer medications
    f. Allay anxiety
    g. Maintain respiratory precautions
    h. Force fluids
    i. Maintain bed rest
    j. Instruct patient to cover nose and mouth when sneezing
    k. Provide frequent oral hygiene
    l. Provide ultraviolet light or well-ventilated room
8. Patient/family teaching goals; the patient will:
    a. Keep follow-up appointments
    b. Stop smoking
    c. Maintain ideal weight
    d. State the action, side effects, and scheduling of medications
    e. Identify and reduce stress
    f. Recognize the signs and symptoms of respiratory infection
    g. Adhere to activity limitations
    h. Avoid exposure to people with infections
    i. Alternate rest periods with activity
    j. Monitor self for infection
    k. Follow dietary recommendations and restrictions
    l. Seek help from community agencies and resources
    m. Demonstrate methods to prevent spread of droplets of sputum
    n. Provide adequate air ventilation in rooms

9. Possible medical complications
    a. Atelectasis
    b. Spontaneous pneumothorax
10. Possible surgical interventions: surgical resection of infected areas
    (lobectomy) (see page 231)

P. Pneumothorax

1. Definition
    a. Loss of negative intrapleural pressure results in collapse of the lung
    b. Types include spontaneous, open, tension
2. Possible etiology
    a. Blunt chest trauma
    b. Rupture of a bleb
    c. Central venous pressure (CVP) line insertion
    d. Thoracentesis
    e. Penetrating chest injuries
3. Pathophysiology
    a. The loss of negative intrapleural pressure causes the collapse of the lung
    b. Surface area for gas exchange is reduced, resulting in hypoxia and
       hypercarbia
    c. Spontaneous pneumothorax occurs with rupture of bleb
    d. Open pneumothorax occurs when an opening through chest wall allows
       entrance of positive atmospheric pressure into pleural space
    e. Tension pneumothorax occurs when there is a buildup of positive
       pressure in the pleural space
4. Possible clinical manifestations
    a. Sharp pain that increases with exertion
    b. Diminished or absent breath sounds unilaterally
    c. Dyspnea
    d. Tracheal shift
    e. Anxiety
    f. Diaphoresis
    g. Tachycardia
    h. Tachypnea
    i. Decreased chest expansion unilaterally
    j. Subcutaneous emphysema
    k. Pallor
    l. Cough
5. Possible diagnostic test findings
    a. CXR: pneumothorax
    b. ABGs: respiratory acidosis, hypoxemia
6. Medical management
    a. Oxygen therapy
    b. Position: high-Fowler
    c. Activity: out of bed to chair, active ROM to affected arm
    d. Monitoring: VS, I/O

    e. Laboratory studies: ABGs

    f. Treatments: incentive spirometry

    g. Insertion of chest tube to water-seal drainage

    h. Thoracentesis

    i. Analgesics: oxycodone hydrochloride (Tylox)

7. Medical nursing interventions/responsibilities

    a. Administer oxygen

    b. Provide pulmonary toilet: TCDB, incentive spirometry

    c. Assess respiratory status

    d. Maintain chest tube to water-seal drainage

    e. Maintain high-Fowler position

    f. Monitor and record VS, chest tube drainage, presence of air leak or subcutaneous emphysema, laboratory studies

    g. Administer medications

    h. Allay anxiety

    i. Assess pain

8. Patient/family teaching goals; the patient will:

    a. Keep follow-up appointments

    b. Stop smoking

    c. State the action, side effects, and scheduling of medications

    d. Recognize the signs and symptoms of pneumothorax and respiratory infection

    e. Avoid heavy lifting

9. Possible medical complications

    a. Mediastinal shift

    b. Respiratory insufficiency

    c. Infection

10. Possible surgical interventions: none

Q. Pulmonary embolism

1. Definition

    a. Presence of an undissolved substance in the pulmonary vasculature that results in obstruction of blood flow

    b. Types: fat, air, thrombus

2. Possible etiology

    a. Flat, long bone fractures

    b. Thrombophlebitis

    c. Venous stasis

    d. Hypercoagulability

    e. Abdominal surgery

    f. Malignant tumors

    g. Prolonged bedrest

    h. Obesity

3. Pathophysiology

    a. Air, fat, or the tail of a thrombus that breaks off travels from the venous circulation to the right side of the heart and pulmonary artery

      b. Blood flow is obstructed by the embolism, resulting in pulmonary hypertension and possible infarction

4. Possible clinical manifestations
   a. Dyspnea
   b. Tachycardia
   c. Elevated temperature
   d. Cough
   e. Hemoptysis
   f. Chest pain
   g. Tachypnea
   h. Anxiety
   i. Rales
   j. Hypotension
   k. Dysrhythmias
5. Possible diagnostic test findings
   a. CXR: dilated pulmonary arteries
   b. ABGs: respiratory alkalosis, hypoxemia
   c. Lung scan: decreased pulmonary circulation, blood flow obstruction
   d. Angiography: location of embolism, filling defect of pulmonary artery
   e. Blood chemistry: increased lactic dehydrogenase (LDH)
   f. EKG: tachycardia, nonspecific ST changes
6. Medical management
   a. I.V. therapy: hydration, heparin lock
   b. Oxygen therapy
   c. Intubation and mechanical ventilation
   d. Position: high-Fowler
   e. Activity: bed rest, active and passive ROM, isometric exercises
   f. Monitoring: VS, UO, CVP, EKG, I/O, neurovascular checks
   g. Laboratory studies: ABGs, PT, PTT
   h. Treatments: Foley catheter, incentive spirometry
   i. Analgesics: meperidine hydrochloride (Demerol)
   j. Diuretics: furosemide (Lasix), ethacrynic acid (Edecin)
   k. Anticoagulants: heparin (Lipo-Hepin), warfarin sodium (Coumadin)
   l. Fibrinolytics: streptokinase, urokinase
7. Medical nursing interventions/responsibilities
   a. Administer I.V. fluids
   b. Administer oxygen
   c. Provide pulmonary toilet: suction, TCDB
   d. Assess respiratory status
   e. Maintain high-Fowler position
   f. Monitor and record VS, UO, CVP, I/O, urine for blood, laboratory studies
   g. Administer medications
   h. Allay anxiety
   i. Monitor color, consistency, and amount of sputum
   j. Assess for positive Homans' sign

8. Patient/family teaching goals; the patient will:
   a. Keep follow-up appointments
   b. Maintain regular exercise program
   c. Stop smoking
   d. Maintain ideal weight
   e. State the action, side effects, and scheduling of medications
   f. Identify and reduce stress
   g. Recognize the signs and symptoms of respiratory distress
   h. Avoid prolonged sitting and standing
   i. Avoid constrictive clothing
   j. Avoid crossing legs when seated
   k. Avoid using oral contraceptives
9. Possible medical complications: pulmonary infarction
10. Possible surgical interventions
   a. Vein ligation
   b. Ligation of inferior vena cava (see page 233)
   c. Embolectomy (see page 232)

R. Lung cancer
1. Definition: malignant tumor of the lung that may be primary or metastatic
2. Possible etiology
   a. Cigarette smoking
   b. Exposure to environmental pollutants
   c. Exposure to occupational pollutants
3. Pathophysiology
   a. Unregulated cell growth and uncontrolled cell division result in the development of a neoplasm
   b. Four histologic types include epidermoid (squamous), adenocarcinoma, large cell anaplastic, small cell anaplastic
   c. Lungs are common target site for metastasis from other organs
4. Possible clinical manifestations
   a. Cough
   b. Dyspnea
   c. Hemoptysis
   d. Chest pain
   e. Chills
   f. Fever
   g. Weight loss
   h. Weakness
   i. Anorexia
   j. Wheezing
   k. Fatigue
5. Possible diagnostic test findings
   a. CXR: lesion or mass
   b. Bronchoscopy: positive biopsy
   c. Angiography: involvement of pulmonary artery or pulmonary veins

      d. Sputum studies: positive cytology for cancer cells

      e. Lung scan: presence of mass

6. Medical management

      a. Diet therapy: high-protein, high-calorie

      b. I.V. therapy: heparin lock

      c. Oxygen therapy

      d. Intubation and mechanical ventilation

      e. Position: semi-Fowler

      f. Actvity: ad lib, active and passive ROM

      g. Monitoring: VS, UO, I/O

      h. Laboratory studies: ABGs

      i. Nutritional support: IVH

      j. Radiation therapy

      k. Antineoplastics: cyclophosphamide (Cytoxan), doxorubicin hydrochloride (Adriamycin)

      l. Treatments: incentive spirometry

      m. Isotope implant

      n. Laser photocoagulation

      o. Diuretics: furosemide (Lasix), ethacrynic acid (Edecrin)

      p. Chemotherapy

7. Medical nursing interventions/responsibilities

      a. Maintain diet

      b. Encourage fluids

      c. Administer I.V. fluids

      d. Administer oxygen

      e. Provide pulmonary toilet: suction, TCDB

      f. Assess respiratory status

      g. Maintain semi-Fowler position

      h. Monitor and record VS, UO, I/O, laboratory studies

      i. Administer IVH

      j. Administer medications

      k. Encourage ventilation of feelings about change in body image, fear of dying

      l. Assess pain

      m. Provide postchemotherapeutic and/or postradiation nursing care: provide skin, mouth, and perineal care; encourage dietary intake; administer antiemetics and antidiarrheals; monitor for bleeding, infection, and electrolyte imbalance; provide rest periods

8. Patient/family teaching goals, the patient will:

      a. Keep follow-up appointments

      b. Maintain regular exercise program

      c. Stop smoking

      d. Maintain ideal weight

      e. State the action, side effects, and scheduling of medications

      f. Demonstrate deep breathing and coughing exercises

g. Alternate rest periods with activity
h. Follow dietary recommendations and restrictions
9. Possible medical complications
    a. Respiratory insufficiency
    b. Pneumonia
10. Possible surgical interventions
    a. Lung resection (see page 231)
    b. Lobectomy (see page 231)
    c. Wedge resection (see page 231)
    d. Pneumonectomy (see page 231)

S. Laryngeal cancer
1. Definition: benign or malignant tumor of the larynx
2. Possible etiology
    a. Cigarette smoking
    b. Alcohol abuse
    c. Exposure to environmental pollutants
    d. Exposure to radiation
    e. Voice strain
3. Pathophysiology
    a. Unregulated cell growth and uncontrolled cell division result in the
        development of a neoplasm through growth of abnormal cells
    b. Most laryngeal cancers are squamous cell carcinomas
    c. Intrinsic cancer is cancer within the larynx
    d. Extrinsic cancer is cancer outside the larynx
4. Possible clinical manifestations
    a. Throat pain
    b. Burning sensation
    c. Palpable lump in neck
    d. Dysphagia
    e. Dyspnea
    f. Cough
    g. Hemoptysis
    h. Progressive hoarseness
    i. Sore throat
    j. Weakness
    k. Weight loss
    l. Foul breath
5. Possible diagnostic test findings
    a. Laryngoscopy: lesions, ulcerations, positive biopsy
    b. Biopsy: cytology positive for cancer cells
6. Medical management
    a. Diet therapy: high-calorie, high-vitamin, high-protein
    b. I.V. therapy: heparin lock
    c. Oxygen therapy

    d. Position: semi-Fowler

    e. Activity: as tolerated

    f. Monitoring: VS, UO, I/O

    g. Laboratory studies: Hgb, Hct, ABGs

    h. Nutritional support: IVH, NG tube feedings, gastrostomy feedings

    i. Radiation therapy

    j. Chemotherapy

    k. Treatments: incentive spirometry

    l. Analgesics: oxycodone hydrochloride (Tylox)

7. Medical nursing interventions/responsibilities

    a. Maintain high-calorie, high-vitamin, high-protein diet

    b. Administer I.V. fluids

    c. Administer oxygen

    d. Provide pulmonary toilet: incentive spirometry, TCDB

    e. Assess respiratory status

    f. Maintain activity as tolerated

    g. Maintain semi-Fowler position

    h. Monitor and record VS, UO, I/O, laboratory studies

    i. Administer IVH, NG tube feedings, gastrostomy feedings

    j. Administer medications

    k. Encourage ventilation of feelings about potential loss of voice and change in body image

    l. Assess color, amount, and consistency of sputum

    m. Provide postchemotherapeutic and/or postradiation nursing care: provide skin, mouth, and perineal care; encourage dietary intake; administer antiemetics and antidiarrheals; monitor for bleeding, infection, and electrolyte imbalance; provide rest periods

8. Patient/family teaching goals; the patient will:

    a. Keep follow-up appointments

    b. Stop smoking

    c. Maintain ideal weight

    d. State the action, side effects, and scheduling of medications

    e. Recognize the signs and symptoms of respiratory distress

    f. Limit use of voice

    g. Avoid exposure to people with infections

    h. Alternate rest periods with activity

    i. Monitor self for infection

    j. Follow dietary recommendations and restrictions

    k. Seek help from community agencies and resources

9. Possible medical complications

    a. Laryngeal obstruction

    b. Respiratory distress

10. Possible surgical interventions

    a. Partial laryngectomy (see page 228)

    b. Total laryngectomy (see page 228)

    c. Radical neck dissection (see page 229)

Points to Remember

Elevate the head of the bed to promote maximum lung expansion to compensate for ventilation deficits in the patient with a respiratory system disorder.

Nursing measures that decrease the patient's anxiety and allay the fear of suffocation will decrease the patient's respiratory effort.

Pulmonary toilet is essential in preventing respiratory complications.

Environmental factors contribute to the exacerbation of respiratory illness symptomatology.

Assessment of patients with respiratory system disorders should include evaluation of compensatory cardiac function.

Glossary

Dyspnea — difficult, labored breathing.

Hemoptysis — expectoration of bloody sputum.

Rales — abnormal inspiratory or expiratory lung sound, usually associated with presence of fluid.

Rhonchi — abnormal inspiratory or expiratory lung sound, usually associated with airway constriction.

Tachypnea — abnormally fast rate of breathing.

Integumentary System

Learning Objectives

After studying this section, the reader should be able to:

- Describe the psychosocial impact of integumentary system disorders.

- Differentiate between modifiable and nonmodifiable risk factors in the development of an integumentary system disorder.

- List three potential and three actual nursing diagnoses for the patient with an integumentary system disorder.

- Identify the medical and surgical nursing interventions/responsibilities for the patient with an integumentary system disorder.

- Write three teaching goals for the patient with an integumentary system disorder.

VIII. Integumentary System

A. Anatomy and physiology

1. Skin: first line of defense against microorganisms; composed of epidermal, dermal, and subcutaneous layers
2. Epidermis
   a. Outer avascular layer composed of dense squamous cells that constantly shed
   b. Keratinocytes and melanocytes in this layer
3. Dermis:
   a. Origin of hair, nails, sebaceous glands, eccrine sweat glands, apocrine sweat glands
   b. Collagen layer that supports epidermis and contains nerves and blood vessels
4. Subcutaneous tissue (hypodermis)
   a. Third layer of skin, composed of loose connective tissue filled with fatty cells
   b. It provides heat, insulation, shock absorption, and a reserve of calories
5. Hair
   a. It protects and covers the body, except for palms, lips, soles of feet, nipples, and external genitalia
   b. Hormones stimulate differential growth
6. Nails
   a. Composed of dead cells filled with keratin
   b. Protect tips of fingers and toes
7. Glandular appendages
   a. Three types are sebaceous, eccrine, and apocrine
   b. Sebaceous glands (oil), which lubricate hair and epidermis, are stimulated by sex hormones
   c. Eccrine sweat glands regulate body temperature through water secretion
   d. Apocrine sweat glands, located in the axilla, nipple, anal, and pubic areas, secrete odorless fluid; decomposition of this fluid by bacteria causes odor

B. Physical assessment findings

1. Subjective data that often accompany integumentary disorders
   a. Change in skin color, texture, and temperature
   b. Perspiration or dryness
   c. Itching
   d. Brittle, thick, or soft nails
   e. Fever
   f. Hair loss
   g. Rash
2. Objective data to evaluate in integumentary disorders
   a. Pattern of pigmentation and hair distribution
   b. Skin texture, turgor, color, and temperature

   c. Peripheral edema
   d. Trophic changes: skin, hair, and nails
   e. Skin lesions: type, shape, and character
   f. Pruritus
   g. Nevi and scars
   h. Elevated body temperature
   i. Erythema
   j. Petechiae and ecchymosis

C. Diagnostic tests and procedures used to evaluate integumentary disorders
   1. Blood chemistry
       a. Definition/purpose: laboratory analysis of blood sample for potassium, sodium, calcium, phosphorus, ketones, glucose, osmolality, chloride, blood urea nitrogen (BUN), and creatinine (Cr)
       b. Nursing interventions/responsibilities: before procedure, withhold food and fluids as ordered; after procedure, assess site for bleeding
   2. Hematologic studies
       a. Definition/purpose: laboratory analysis of blood sample for red blood cells (RBC), white blood cells (WBC), erythrocyte sedimentation rate (ESR), platelets, prothrombin time (PT), partial thromboplastin time (PTT), hemoglobin (Hgb), hematocrit (Hct)
       b. Nursing interventions/responsibilities: assess site for bleeding
   3. Skin biopsy (punch biopsy)
       a. Definition/purpose: removal of a small amount of skin tissue for histologic evaluation using a circular punch instrument
       b. Nursing interventions/responsibilities: assess site for bleeding and infection
   4. Skin testing
       a. Definition/purpose: administration of allergen to the skin's surface or into the dermis through patch, scratch, or intradermal technique
       b. Nursing interventions/responsibilities: keep area dry; record site, date, and time of test; assess site for erythema, papules, vesicles, edema, and induration; record date and time for follow-up site reading
   5. Skin scrapings
       a. Definition/purpose: microscopic examination of scales, nails, and hair that have been scraped by a scalpel and covered with potassium hydroxide
       b. Nursing interventions/responsibilities: assess site for bleeding and infection
   6. Skin studies
       a. Definition/purpose: microscopic examination of skin, including gram stain, culture and sensitivity, cytology, and immunofluorescence (IF)
       b. Nursing interventions/responsibilities: follow laboratory procedure guidelines; note current antibiotic therapy
   7. Wood's light
       a. Definition/purpose: direct examination of skin using ultraviolet (UV) light
       b. Nursing interventions/responsibilities: explain procedure; allay anxiety

D. Possible psychosocial impact of integumentary disorders
1. Developmental impact
   a. Change in body image
   b. Fear of rejection
   c. Change in role performance
   d. Decreased self-esteem
2. Economic impact
   a. Cost of cosmetics
   b. Disruption or loss of employment
   c. Cost of hospitalizations and follow-up care
   d. Cost of medications
3. Occupational and recreational impact
   a. Restrictions in physical activity
   b. Change in leisure activity
4. Social impact
   a. Social isolation
   b. Sexual dysfunction

E. Possible risk factors for integumentary disorders
1. Modifiable risk factors
   a. Infection
   b. Occupation
   c. Exposure to chemical and environmental pollutants
   d. Exposure to radiation
   e. Exposure to sun
   f. Personal hygiene habits
   g. Climate
   h. Use of cosmetics and soaps
   i. Stress
   j. Nutritional deficiencies
   k. Medications
   l. Crowded living conditions
2. Nonmodifiable risk factors
   a. Aging process
   b. History of endocrine, vascular, or immune disorders
   c. Family history of skin disease or allergies
   d. History of allergies
   e. Exposure to communicable disease
   f. Pregnancy
   g. Menopause

F. Possible nursing diagnoses for the patient with integumentary disorders
1. Actual nursing diagnoses
   a. Impairment of skin integrity
   b. Disturbance of self-concept: body image
   c. Disturbance of self-concept: self-esteem

   d. Alteration in comfort: pain
   e. Sensory-perceptual alteration: tactile
2. Potential nursing diagnoses
   a. Ineffective breathing patterns
   b. Ineffective individual coping
   c. Fluid volume deficit
   d. Potential for injury: infection
   e. Anxiety
   f. Social isolation

G. Surgical intervention: skin graft
   1. Definition
      a. Replacement of damaged skin with healthy skin to protect underlying
          structures or to reconstruct areas for cosmetic or functional purposes
      b. Split-thickness graft: graft of half of the epidermis, which is removed by
          a dermatome
      c. Full-thickness graft: graft of the entire epidermis
      d. Pinch graft: graft of a small piece of skin, obtained by elevating the skin
          with a needle and removing it with scissors
   2. Preoperative surgical nursing interventions/responsibilities
      a. Complete patient and family preoperative teaching: assess their
          understanding of surgical procedure; explain operating room (OR),
          recovery room (RR), preoperative and postoperative routine; demonstrate
          postoperative turning, coughing, and deep breathing (TCDB), splinting,
          leg exercises, and range-of-motion (ROM) exercises; explain
          postoperative need for drainage tubes, surgical dressings, oxygen therapy,
          I.V. therapy, and pain control
      b. Complete preoperative check list
      c. Administer preoperative medications
      d. Allay patient and family anxiety about surgery
      e. Document patient history and physical assesssment data base
      f. Prepare donor and recipient site
   3. Postoperative surgical nursing interventions/responsibilities
      a. Assess pain and administer postoperative analgesic
      b. Progress diet as tolerated
      c. Administer I.V. fluids
      d. Allay anxiety
      e. Provide hydrotherapy as ordered
      f. Reinforce TCDB
      g. Assess for return of peristalsis
      h. Provide pulmonary toilet: incentive spirometry
      i. Maintain activity: as tolerated, active and passive ROM, isometric
          exercises
      j. Avoid weight bearing on extremity with recipient site
      k. Monitor vital signs (VS), urinary output (UO), intake and output (I/O),
          neurovascular checks distal to recipient site

     l. Elevate and immobilize recipient sites
     m. Encourage ventilation of feelings about change in body image
     n. Administer antibiotics
     o. Assess recipient site for infection, hematoma, and fluid accumulation under the graft
     p. Keep donor site dry
     q. Prevent scratching
     r. Apply heat lamp to donor site

4. Possible surgical complications
     a. Infection of recipient and donor sites
     b. Graft rejection or failure
     c. Hematoma under graft
     d. Fluid accumulation under graft

5. Patient/family postoperative teaching goals; the patient will:
     a. Keep follow-up appointments
     b. Maintain regular exercise program
     c. Stop smoking
     d. Maintain ideal weight
     e. State the action, side effects, and scheduling of medications
     f. Recognize the signs and symptoms of infection
     g. Continue physical therapy
     h. Apply lubricating lotion to recipient site
     i. Protect recipient site from direct sunlight
     j. Avoid trauma to recipient site
     k. Avoid extreme temperatures
     l. Demonstrate cosmetic camouflage techniques
     m. Complete daily dressing changes

H. Contact dermatitis

1. Definition: inflammatory response of the skin after contact with a specific antigen
2. Possible etiology
     a. Mechanical, biological, and chemical irritants
     b. Cosmetics and hair dyes
     c. Detergents, cleaning agents, soaps
     d. Insecticides
     e. Poison ivy
     f. Wool
3. Pathophysiology
     a. Contact with an antigen triggers a localized inflammatory response
     b. Inflammatory response produces skin changes
4. Possible clinical manifestations
     a. Pruritus and burning
     b. Erythema at point of contact
     c. Localized edema
     d. Vesicles and papules

    e. Lichenification
    f. Pigmentation changes
    g. Eczema
    h. Scaling
5. Possible diagnostic test findings
    a. Skin test (patch): positive to specific antigen
    b. Visual examination: area of dermatitis correlates with area of antigen contact
6. Medical management
    a. Position: elevation of extremity
    b. Activity: as tolerated
    c. Monitoring: VS, neurovascular checks
    d. Treatments: cool, wet dressings with aluminum acetate solution (Burow's solution) tepid baths, bed cradle
    e. Antibiotics: ampicillin (Omnipen)
    f. Antipruritics: diphenhydramine hydrochloride (Benadryl)
    g. Corticosteroids: hydrocortisone (Cort-done)
    h. Antihistamines: diphenhydramine hydrochloride (Benadryl)
    i. Antianxiety agents: diazepam (Valium)
7. Medical nursing interventions/responsibilities
    a. Assess neurovascular status
    b. Maintain elevation of affected extremity
    c. Monitor and record VS and neurovascular checks
    d. Administer medications
    e. Encourage ventilation of feelings about change in physical appearance
    f. Provide treatments: tepid baths; bed cradle; cool, wet dressings
    g. Avoid soaps
    h. Avoid use of heating pads or blankets
    i. Avoid temperature extremes
    j. Prevent scratching and rubbing of affected area
    k. Maintain a cool environment
    l. Provide diversional activities
8. Patient/family teaching goals; the patient will:
    a. Keep follow-up appointments
    b. Stop smoking
    c. State the action, side effects, and scheduling of medications
    d. Recognize the signs and symptoms of infection
    e. Monitor self for infection
    f. Avoid causative agent
    g. Avoid skin dryness, soaps, and heat
    h. Avoid the use of over-the-counter medication
    i. Protect affected area from trauma, excessive sunlight, wind, and temperature extremes
    j. Avoid scratching and rubbing of affected areas
9. Possible medical complications: infection
10. Possible surgical interventions: none

I. **Psoriasis**
   1. Definition: chronic, noninfectious skin inflammation that occurs in patches
   2. Possible etiology
      a. Stress
      b. Epidermal trauma
      c. Streptococcal infection
      d. Change in climate
      e. Genetics
      f. Anxiety
      g. Alcoholism
      h. Rheumatoid arthritis
      i. Drug induced: lithium, propranolol
      j. Hormones
      k. Obesity
   3. Pathophysiology
      a. Loss of normal regulatory mechanisms of cell division leads to rapid multiplication of epidermal cells that interferes with formation of normal protective layer of skin
      b. Papules coalesce to form plaques
   4. Possible clinical manifestations
      a. Pruritus
      b. Shedding, scaling plaques
      c. Yellow discoloration and thickening of nails
      d. Erythema
      e. Papules on sacrum, nails, palms
   5. Possible diagnostic test findings: plaques, on visual examination
   6. Medical management
      a. Monitoring: VS, neurovascular checks
      b. Treatments: bed cradle, daily soaks, and tepid, wet compresses
      c. Corticosteroids: triamcinolone (Kenalog) covered with occlusive dressing
      d. Antipsoriatics: anthralin (Anthra-Derm), coal tar (Estar), followed by exposure to UV light
      e. Antimetabolites: methotrexate (Amethopterin)
      f. Photochemotherapy (PUVA therapy): methoxsalen (Psoralen) followed by exposure to black light
      g. Keratolytics: benzoyl peroxide (Benzagel), salicylic acid (Klaron)
   7. Medical nursing interventions/responsibilities
      a. Assess neurovascular status
      b. Monitor and record VS, neurovascular checks
      c. Administer medications
      d. Encourage ventilation of feelings about change in body image
      e. Administer UV light and PUVA therapy
      f. Apply occlusive dressings
      g. Prevent scratching
      h. Help patient to remove scales during soaks

8. Patient/family teaching goals; the patient will:
   a. Keep follow-up appointments
   b. Stop smoking
   c. Maintain ideal weight
   d. State the action, side effects, and scheduling of medications
   e. Identify and reduce stress
   f. Recognize the signs and symptoms of infection
   g. Wear light cotton clothing over affected areas
   h. Avoid over-the-counter medications
   i. Demonstrate dressing change
   j. Complete daily skin care
   k. Protect affected area from trauma
9. Possible medical complications
   a. Depression
   b. Infection
   c. Rheumatoid arthritis
10. Possible surgical interventions: none

J. Herpes zoster (shingles)
1. Definition: acute viral infection of nerve structure caused by varicella zoster
2. Possible etiology
   a. Cytotoxic drug-induced immunosuppression
   b. Hodgkin's disease
   c. Exposure to varicella zoster
   d. Debilitating disease
3. Pathophysiology
   a. Activation of dormant varicella zoster virus causes an inflammatory reaction
   b. Affected areas include spinal and cranial sensory ganglia and posterior gray matter of the spinal cord
4. Possible clinical manifestations
   a. Neuralgia
   b. Malaise
   c. Pruritus
   d. Burning
   e. Unilaterally clustered skin vesicles along peripheral sensory nerves on trunk, thorax, or face
   f. Erythema
   g. Fever
   h. Anorexia
   i. Headache
   j. Parasthesia
   k. Edematous skin

5. Possible diagnostic test findings
    a. Antinuclear antibody (ANA): positive
    b. Skin cultures and stains: identification of organism
    c. Visual examination: vesicles along peripheral sensory nerves
6. Medical management
    a. Activity: as tolerated
    b. Monitoring: VS, seventh cranial nerve function, neurovascular checks
    c. Treatments: air mattress, acetic acid compresses, tepid baths, bed cradle
    d. Analgesics: acetaminophen (Tylenol), oxycodone hydrochloride (Tylox)
    e. Antianxiety agents: diazepam (Valium), hydroxyzine (Vistaril)
    f. Antipruritics: diphenhydramine hydrochloride (Benadryl)
    g. Corticosteroids: hydrocortisone (Cortef), triamcinolone acetonide (Kenalog)
    h. Nerve block using lidocaine (Xylocaine)
    i. Antiviral agents: acycloguanosine (Acyclovir), vidarabine (Vira-A), interferon
    j. Laboratory studies: culture and sensitivity
7. Medical nursing interventions/responsibilities
    a. Assess pain
    b. Monitor and record VS, laboratory results, seventh cranial nerve function
    c. Administer medications as ordered
    d. Encourage ventilation of feelings about change in physical appearance and recurrent nature of illness
    e. Provide treatments: acetic acid compresses, tepid baths, bed cradle, air mattress
    f. Prevent scratching and rubbing of affected area
    g. Allay anxiety
8. Patient/family teaching goals; the patient will:
    a. Keep follow-up appointments
    b. Stop smoking
    c. State the action, side effects, and scheduling of medications
    d. Recognize the signs and symptoms of infection and hearing loss
    e. Monitor self for infection
    f. Avoid wool and synthetic clothing
    g. Wear lightweight, loose cotton clothing
    h. Keep blisters intact
    i. Avoid scratching and rubbing affected areas
9. Possible medical complications
    a. Infection
    b. Postherpetic neuralgia
    c. Ophthalmic herpes zoster
    d. Facial paralysis
    e. Vertigo

    f. Tinnitus
    g. Hearing loss
    h. Visceral dissemination
  10. Possible surgical interventions: none

K. Burns
  1. Definition: destruction of epidermis, dermis, and subcutaneous layers of skin
  2. Possible etiology
    a. Radiation: X-ray, sun, nuclear reactors
    b. Mechanical: friction
    c. Chemical: acids, alkalies, vesicants
    d. Electrical: lightning, electrical wires
    e. Thermal: flame, frostbite, scald
  3. Pathophysiology
    a. Cell destruction causes loss of intracellular fluid and electrolytes
    b. Amount of cell destruction is directly related to extent (area) and degree (depth) of burn
    c. First-degree (superficial partial thickness) involves epidermal layer
    d. Second-degree (dermal partial thickness) involves epidermal and dermal layers
    e. Third-degree (full thickness) involves epidermal, dermal, subcutaneous layers, and nerve endings
  4. Possible clinical manifestations
    a. First-degree: erythema, edema, pain, blanching
    b. Second-degree: pain; oozing, fluid-filled vesicles; erythema; shiny, wet subcutaneous layer after vesicles rupture
    c. Third-degree: Eschar, edema, little or no pain
  5. Possible diagnostic test findings
    a. Blood chemistry: increased potassium; decreased sodium, albumin, complement fixation, immunoglobulins
    b. Arterial blood gases (ABGs): metabolic acidosis
    c. 24-hour urine collection: decreased creatinine clearance, negative nitrogen balance
    d. Hematology: increased Hgb, Hct; decreased fibrinogen, platelets, WBC
    e. Urine chemistry: hematuria, myoglobinuria
    f. Visual examination: extent of burn determined by Rule of Nines
  6. Medical management
    a. Diet therapy: high-protein, high-fat, high-calorie, high-carbohydrate, in small, frequent feedings; withhold food and fluids
    b. I.V. therapy: hydration and electrolyte replacement using Evan, Brooke, Parkland, or Massachusetts General Hospital protocols; heparin lock
    c. Oxygen therapy
    d. Intubation and mechanical ventilation
    e. Gastrointestinal decompression: nasogastric (NG) tube, Miller-Abbott tube
    f. Position: semi-Fowler

  g. Activity: bed rest
  h. Monitoring: VS, UO, EKG, hemodynamic variables, I/O, neurovital signs, neurovascular checks, stool for occult blood
  i. Laboratory studies: potassium, sodium, glucose, osmolality, Cr, BUN, Hgb, Hct, platelets, WBC, ABGs, culture and sensitivity
  j. Nutritional support: I.V. hyperalimentation (IVH), NG feedings
  k. Treatments: Foley catheter, postural drainage, chest physiotherapy (CPT), incentive spirometry, bed cradle, intermittent positive pressure breathing (IPPB), suction, Jobst clothing, Hubbard tank bath
  l. Precautions: protective
  m. Transfusion therapy: fresh frozen plasma (FFP), platelets, packed red blood cells (PRBC), plasma
  n. Antibiotics: gentamicin sulfate (Garamycin)
  o. Anti-infectives: mafenide (Sulfamylon), silver sulfadiazine (Silvadene), silver nitrate, povidone-iodine (Betadine)
  p. Antianxiety: diazepam (Valium)
  q. Antitetanus: tetanus toxoid
  r. Analgesic: morphine sulfate (Roxanol)
  s. Antacids: magnesium and aluminum hydroxide (Maalox), aluminum hydroxide gel (Alternagel)
  t. Histamine antagonists: cimetidine (Tagamet), ranitidine (Zantac)
  u. Vitamins: phytonadione (AquaMEPHYTON), cyanocobalamine (vitamin B_{12})
  v. Colloids: 5% albumin (Albuminar)
  w. Diuretics: mannitol (Osmitrol)
  x. Sedatives: phenobarbital (Luminal)
  y. Cardiac glycosides: digoxin (Lanoxin)
  z. Escharotomy
7. Medical nursing interventions/responsibilities
  a. Maintain diet; withhold food and fluids
  b. Administer I.V. fluids
  c. Administer oxygen
  d. Provide pulmonary toilet: suction, TCDB, IPPB, CPT, postural drainage
  e. Assess respiratory status and fluid balance
  f. Assess pain
  g. Maintain position, patency, low suction of NG tube
  h. Maintain semi-Fowler position
  i. Monitor and record VS, UO, I/O, laboratory studies, hemodynamic variables, neurovital signs, stool for occult blood, specific gravity, calorie count, daily weight, neurovascular checks
  j. Provide tracheostomy care or endotube care
  k. Administer IVH
  l. Administer medications
  m. Encourage ventilation of feelings about immobility from scarring, disfigurement, fear of dying

n. Allay anxiety
o. Provide treatments: ROM, tanking, bed cradle, splints, Jobst clothing
p. Alternate periods of rest with activity
q. Elevate affected extremities
r. Maintain a warm environment during acute period
s. Maintain protective precautions
t. Provide skin and mouth care
u. Assess bowel sounds
8. Patient/family teaching goals; the patient will:
  a. Keep follow-up appointments
  b. Maintain regular exercise program
  c. Stop smoking
  d. Maintain ideal weight
  e. State the action, side effects, and scheduling of medications
  f. Identify and reduce stress
  g. Recognize the signs and symptoms of infection
  h. Alternate periods of rest with activity
  i. Monitor self for infection
  j. Follow dietary recommendations and restrictions
  k. Complete daily skin care
  l. Demonstrate dressing changes
  m. Avoid trauma to affected area
  n. Avoid restrictive clothing
  o. Avoid fabric softeners, harsh detergents, and soaps
  p. Lubricate healing skin with cocoa butter
  q. Maintain a cool environment
  r. Protect affected area from sunlight
  s. Use splints and Jobst clothing
9. Possible medical complications
  a. Paralytic ileus
  b. Curling's ulcer
  c. Acute renal failure
  d. Pneumonia
  e. Congestive heart failure
  f. Septicemia
  g. Pulmonary edema
10. Possible surgical interventions: skin grafting (see page 254)

L. Skin cancer
1. Definition
  a. Malignant primary tumor of the epidermal layer of the skin
  b. Types: basal cell epithelioma, melanoma, and squamous cell carcinoma
2. Possible etiology
  a. Heredity
  b. Chemical irritants
  c. Ultraviolet rays

     d. Radiation
     e. Friction or chronic irritation
     f. Immunosuppressive drugs
     g. Precancerous lesions: leukoplakia, nevi, senile keratoses
     h. Infrared heat or light
3. Pathophysiology
     a. Unregulated cell growth and uncontrolled cell division result in the development of a neoplasm
     b. Basal cell epithelioma: basal cell keratinization causes tumor growth in basal layer of the epidermis
     c. Melanoma: tumor arises from melanocytes of the epidermis
     d. Squamous cell carcinoma: tumor arises from keratinocytes
4. Possible clinical manifestations
     a. Basal cell epithelioma: waxy nodule with telangiectasis
     b. Melanoma: irregular, circular bordered lesion with hues of tan, black, or blue
     c. Squamous cell carcinoma: small, red, nodular lesion that begins as an erythematous macule or plaque with indistinct margins
     d. Pruritus
     e. Local soreness
     f. Change in color, size, or shape of preexisting lesion
     g. Oozing, bleeding, crusting lesion
5. Possible diagnostic test findings (skin biopsy): cytology positive for cancer cells
6. Medical management
     a. I.V. therapy: heparin lock
     b. Monitoring: VS
     c. Radiation therapy
     d. Cryosurgery with liquid nitrogen
     e. Chemosurgery with zinc chloride
     f. Curettage and electrodesiccation
     g. Immunotherapy for melanoma: bacille Calmette-Guérin (BCG) vaccine
     h. Alkalating agents: carmustine (BCNU), dacarbazine (DTIC)
     i. Antineoplastics: hydroxyurea (Hydrea), vincristine sulfate (Oncovin)
     j. Antimetabolites: fluorouracil (5-FU)
7. Medical nursing interventions/responsibilities
     a. Monitor and record VS
     b. Administer medications
     c. Encourage ventilation of feelings about change in body image and fear of dying
     d. Provide postchemotherapeutic and/or postradiation nursing care: provide skin, mouth, and perineal care; encourage dietary intake; administer antiemetics and antidiarrheals; monitor for bleeding, infection, and electrolyte imbalance; provide rest periods
     e. Assess lesions

8. Patient/family teaching goals; the patient will:
   a. Keep follow-up appointments
   b. State the action, side effects, and scheduling of medications
   c. Recognize the signs and symptoms of infection
   d. Avoid exposure to people with infections
   e. Alternate periods of rest with activity
   f. Monitor self for infection
   g. Seek help from community agencies and resources
   h. Avoid contact with chemical irritants
   i. Use sun-screening lotions and layered clothing
   j. Monitor self for lesions that do not heal or that change characteristics
   k. Have moles removed that are subject to chronic irritation
9. Possible medical complications: metastasis (melanoma)
10. Possible surgical interventions
    a. Surgical excision of tumor
    b. Melanoma: bone marrow transplant (see page 273)

Points to Remember

Damage to the epidermis compromises the body's first line of defense against bacterial invasion.

Secondary infection is a common complication of integumentary disorders.

The embarrassment that occurs from changes in skin appearance can result in social isolation for patients.

Because there are many modifiable risk factors for the patient with integumentary system disorders, the patient can often prevent recurrence of the disorders.

Patients with integumentary system disorders are often treated in outpatient settings.

Glossary

Lichenification — thickening and hardening of the epidermis.

Nevi — mole or birthmark.

Pruritus — itching.

Trophic — skin changes that include thickening, drying, and loss of hair caused by prolonged ischemia and malnutrition of tissues.

Vesicle — fluid-filled sac.

Hematolymphatic System

Learning Objectives

After studying this section, the reader should be able to:

- Describe the psychosocial impact of hematolymphatic system disorders.

- Differentiate between modifiable and nonmodifiable risk factors in the development of a hematolymphatic system disorder.

- List three potential and three actual nursing diagnoses for the patient with a hematolymphatic system disorder.

- Identify the medical and surgical nursing interventions/responsibilities for the patient with a hematolymphatic system disorder.

- Write three teaching goals for the patient with a hematolymphatic system disorder.

IX. Hematolymphatic System

A. Anatomy and physiology

1. Lymphatic vessels
   a. Consist of capillary-like structures that are permeable to large molecules
   b. Prevent edema by moving fluid and proteins from interstitial spaces to venous circulation
   c. Reabsorb fats from the small intestine
2. Lymph nodes
   a. Tissue that filters out bacteria and other foreign cells
   b. Regional grouping of lymph nodes: cervicofacial, supraclavicular, axillary, epitrochlear, inguinal, and femoral
3. Lymph
   a. Fluid found in interstitial spaces
   b. Composition: water and end products of cell metabolism
4. Spleen
   a. Is largest lymphatic organ; filters blood, traps formed particles, and destroys bacteria
   b. Serves as blood reservoir
   c. Forms lymphocytes and monocytes
5. Erythrocytes: red blood cells (RBCs)
   a. Formed in the bone marrow; contain hemoglobin (Hgb)
   b. Oxygen binds with Hgb to form oxyhemoglobin
6. Thrombocytes (platelets)
   a. Formed in the bone marrow
   b. Function in the coagulation of blood
7. Leukocytes: white blood cells (WBCs)
   a. Formed in bone marrow and lymphatic tissue; include granulocytes and agranulocytes
   b. Provide immunity and protection from infection by phagocytosis
8. Plasma
   a. Liquid portion of blood
   b. Composition: water, protein (albumin and globulin), glucose, and electrolytes
9. ABO blood groups
   a. System of antigens located on the surface of RBCs that determines blood type
   b. Blood types: A antigen, B antigen, AB antigens, O (zero) antigens
   c. Universal donor: blood type O
   d. Universal recipient: blood type AB
10. Coagulation
    a. Process of blood clotting
    b. Series of reactions involving the conversion of prothrombin to thrombin to fibrinogen to fibrin to form a clot

11. Bone marrow
   a. Two types exist: red and yellow
   b. Hematopoeisis is carried out by red marrow
   c. Hematopoeisis produces erythrocytes, leukocytes, and thrombocytes
   d. Red bone marrow is a source of lymphocytes and macrophages
   e. Yellow bone marrow is red bone marrow that has changed to fat
12. Liver
   a. Is largest organ in the body
   b. Produces bile (main function), which emulsifies fats and stimulates peristalsis
   c. Conveys bile to the duodenum at the sphincter of Oddi through the common bile duct
   d. Metabolizes carbohydrates, fats, and proteins
   e. Synthesizes coagulation factors VII, IX, X, and prothrombin
   f. Stores vitamins A, D, B_{12}, and iron
   g. Detoxifies chemicals
   h. Excretes bilirubin
   i. Receives dual blood supply from portal vein and hepatic artery
   j. Produces and stores glycogen
   k. Promotes erythropoiesis when bone marrow production is insufficient

B. **Physical assessment findings**
   1. Subjective data that often accompany hematolymphatic disorders
      a. Enlarged glands
      b. Pain
      c. Fatigue and weakness
      d. Bleeding
      e. Pallor
      f. Lassitude
      g. Shortness of breath
      h. Fainting
      i. Vertigo
      j. Jaundice
      k. Night sweats
      l. Fever
      m. Weight loss
      n. Tachycardia
      o. Activity intolerance
      p. Frequent infections
      q. Melena
      r. Headache
   2. Objective data to evaluate in hematolymphatic disorders
      a. Lymph node enlargement
      b. Anemia
      c. Ecchymosis
      d. Inspection of skin: pallor, cyanosis, jaundice, petechiae

    e. Gingivitis
    f. Ophthalmoscopic exam: bleeding fundi
    g. Sclera: jaundice, capillary hemorrhage
    h. Hepatomegaly
    i. Sternal tenderness
    j. Splenomegaly
    k. Myocardial hypertrophy
    l. Epistaxis
    m. Dyspnea on exertion

C. **Diagnostic tests and procedures used to evaluate hematolymphatic disorders**
    1. Blood chemistry
        a. Definition/purpose: laboratory analysis of blood sample for potassium, calcium, blood urea nitrogen (BUN), creatinine (Cr), protein, albumin, bilirubin
        b. Nursing interventions/responsibilities: before procedure, withhold food and fluids as ordered; after procedure, monitor site for bleeding
    2. Hematologic studies
        a. Definition/purpose: laboratory analysis of blood sample for WBC, RBC, platelets, prothrombin time (PT), partial thromboplastin time (PTT), erythrocyte sedimentation rate (ESR), Hgb, hematocrit (Hct)
        b. Nursing interventions/responsibilities: assess site for bleeding, note current drug therapy
    3. Lymphangiography
        a. Definition/purpose: radiographic picture of lymphatic system and dissection of lymph vessel after injection of radiopaque dye through a catheter
        b. Nursing interventions/responsibilities: before procedure, assess allergies to radiopaque dyes, iodine, and seafood; inform patient he may feel flushing of the face and throat irritation; obtain written, informed consent; withhold food and fluids as ordered; after procedure, assess vital signs (VS) and peripheral pulses; inspect catheter insertion site for bleeding; force fluids; advise patient that skin, stool, and urine will have blue discoloration
    4. Bone marrow examination (aspiration or biopsy)
        a. Definition/purpose: percutaneous removal of bone marrow to examine erythrocytes, leukocytes, and thrombocytes
        b. Nursing interventions/responsibilities: before procedure, obtain written, informed consent; assess patient's ability to lie still during aspiration; after procedure, maintain pressure dressing; assess site for bleeding and infection
    5. Schilling test
        a. Definition/purpose: microscopic examination of 24-hour urine sample for cyanocobalamin (vitamin B_{12}) after administration of oral radioactive cyanocobalamin and intramuscular cyanocobalamin

b. Nursing interventions/responsibilities: before procedure, withhold food and fluids after midnight; obtain written, informed consent; after procedure, instruct patient to save all voided urine for 24 hours; urine may be kept at room temperature

6. Gastric analysis
   a. Definition/purpose: fasting analysis of gastric secretions by aspirating stomach contents through a nasogastric (NG) tube to measure acidity and diagnose pernicious anemia
   b. Nursing interventions/responsibilities: before procedure, withhold food and fluids, instruct patient not to smoke for 8 to 12 hours before the test; withhold medications that can affect gastric secretions; after procedure, obtain vital signs and assess for reactions to gastric acid stimulant if used

7. Urine urobilinogen
   a. Definition/purpose: microscopic examination of 2-hour or 24-hour urine sample to diagnose hemolytic jaundice
   b. Nursing interventions/responsibilities: use bottle with a preservative and refrigerate specimen; note salicylate use; start urine collection in the afternoon when food is being digested for 2-hour specimen

8. Erythrocyte life span determination
   a. Definition/purpose: measurement of life span of circulating RBCs after reinjection of patient's blood that has been tagged with chromium 51
   b. Nursing interventions/responsibilities: before the procedure, inform patient that frequent blood samples will be drawn over a 2-week period; after procedure, assess injection site for bleeding and apply pressure dressing

9. Bence-Jones protein assay
   a. Definition/purpose: microscopic examination of 24-hour urine collection for the Bence-Jones protein to diagnose multiple myeloma
   b. Nursing interventions/responsibilities: withhold all medications for 48 hours before test; instruct patient to void and note time (collection of urine starts with the next voiding); place urine container on ice; measure each voided urine; instruct patient to void at end of 24-hour period; note medications that might interfere with test

10. Romberg test
    a. Definition/purpose: physical examination to assess loss of balance in pernicious anemia
    b. Nursing interventions/responsibilities: explain the procedure; monitor for imbalance and prevent the patient from falling

11. Erythrocyte fragility test
    a. Definition/purpose: laboratory analysis of blood sample to measure the rate at which RBCs burst in varied hypotonic solutions
    b. Nursing interventions/responsibilities: explain the procedure; send the specimen to the laboratory

12. Rumpel-Leede capillary fragility tourniquet test
    a. Definition/purpose: crude physical examination of vascular resistance, platelet number, and function

       b. Nursing interventions/responsibilities: explain that a blood pressure cuff will be placed on the arm for 5 minutes, followed by counting of petechiae

13. Bone scan
       a. Definition/purpose: visual imaging of bone metabolism after I.V. injection of radioisotope
       b. Nursing interventions/responsibilities: before procedure, assess patient's ability to lie still

D. Possible psychosocial impact of hematolymphatic disorders
1. Developmental impact
       a. Fear of dying
       b. Decreased self-esteem
       c. Fear of rejection
2. Economic impact
       a. Disruption or loss of employment
       b. Cost of hospitalization
       c. Cost of medications
3. Occupational and recreational impact
       a. Restriction in work activity
       b. Change in leisure activity
4. Social impact
       a. Change in role performance
       b. Social isolation

E. Possible risk factors for development of hematolymphatic disorders
1. Modifiable risk factors
       a. Exposure to chemical and environmental pollutants
       b. Sexual activity patterns
       c. History of aspirin use
       d. Alcohol consumption
       e. Drug toxicity
       f. Diet
       g. Exposure to occupational radiation or radiation therapy
2. Nonmodifiable risk factors
       a. Ethnic background
       b. Aging process
       c. Malabsorption syndromes
       d. History of liver disease
       e. History of malignancy

F. Possible nursing diagnoses for the patient with a hematolymphatic disorder
1. Actual nursing diagnoses
       a. Activity intolerance
       b. Ineffective breathing pattern

      c. Alteration in comfort: pain
      d. Impaired gas exchange
  2. Potential nursing diagnoses
      a. Potential for injury: infection
      b. Alteration in nutrition: less than body requirements
      c. Alteration in oral mucous membranes
      d. Disturbance in self-concept: body image
      e. Disturbance in self-concept: self-esteem
      f. Anxiety
      g. Social isolation
      h. Impairment of skin integrity

G. Surgical intervention: splenectomy

  1. Definition: surgical removal of the spleen
  2. Preoperative surgical nursing interventions/responsibilities
      a. Complete patient and family preoperative teaching: assess understanding of surgical procedure; explain operating room (OR), recovery room (RR), preoperative and postoperative routine; demonstrate postoperative turning, coughing, and deep breathing (TCDB), splinting, leg exercises, and range-of-motion (ROM) exercises; explain postoperative need for drainage tubes, surgical dressings, oxygen therapy, I.V. therapy, and pain control
      b. Complete preoperative check list
      c. Administer preoperative medications
      d. Allay patient and family anxiety about surgery
      e. Document patient history and physical assessment data base
      f. Monitor PT, PTT, and platelet count
      g. Administer vitamin K
      h. Verify inoculation with polyvalent pneumococcal vaccine 2 weeks before procedure
      i. Administer antibiotics
  3. Postoperative surgical nursing interventions/responsibilities
      a. Assess cardiac, respiratory, and neurologic status
      b. Assess pain and administer postoperative analgesic
      c. Progress diet as tolerated
      d. Administer I.V. fluids, I.V. hyperalimentation (IVH), and transfusion therapy
      e. Allay anxiety
      f. Assess surgical dressing and change as directed
      g. Reinforce TCDB and splinting of incision
      h. Maintain semi-Fowler position
      i. Assess for return of peristalsis
      j. Provide pulmonary toilet: incentive spirometry
      k. Progress activity as tolerated
      l. Monitor VS, urinary output (UO), intake and output (I/O), laboratory studies

      m. Monitor and maintain position and patency of drainage tubes: wound drainage

      n. Apply abdominal binder

      o. Monitor for abdominal distention

  4. Possible surgical complications

      a. Pneumococcal pneumonia

      b. Infection

      c. Hemorrhage

      d. Sepsis

      e. Disseminated intravascular coagulation (DIC)

      f. Atelectasis

      g. Subphrenic abscess

      h. Thrombophlebitis

  5. Patient/family postoperative teaching goals; the patient will:

      a. Keep follow-up appointments

      b. Maintain regular exercise program

      c. Stop smoking

      d. Maintain ideal weight

      e. State the action, side effects, and scheduling of medications

      f. Recognize the signs and symptoms of infection

      g. Avoid exposure to people with infections

      h. Complete daily incision care

      i. State need for prophylactic use of antibiotics

      j. Avoid contact sports

H. Surgical intervention: bone marrow transplant

  1. Definition

      a. Bone marrow is aspirated from multiple sites along iliac crest of donor

      b. Donor bone marrow is infused intravenously into recipient

  2. Preoperative surgical nursing interventions/responsibilities

      a. Complete patient and family preoperative teaching: assess understanding of surgical procedure; explain OR, RR, preoperative and postoperative routine; demonstrate postoperative TCDB, splinting, leg exercises, and ROM; explain postoperative need for drainage tubes, surgical dressings, oxygen therapy, I.V. therapy, and pain control

      b. Complete preoperative check list

      c. Administer preoperative medications

      d. Allay patient and family anxiety about surgery

      e. Document patient history and physical assessment data base

      f. Verify bone marrow compatibility

      g. Administer chemotherapy for 3 days before transplant

      h. Maintain radiation treatment schedule

      i. Maintain protective isolation or use of laminar air flow room

      j. Monitor for infection

3. Postoperative surgical nursing interventions/responsibilities
    a. Assess cardiac and respiratory status
    b. Progress diet as tolerated
    c. Administer I.V. fluids
    d. Allay anxiety
    e. Assess surgical dressing and change as directed
    f. Maintain semi-Fowler position
    g. Maintain activity as tolerated
    h. Monitor VS, UO, I/O, central venous pressure (CVP), laboratory studies, urine, stool, and emesis for occult blood, daily weight, specific gravity, urine glucose, ketones, and protein
    i. Precautions: protective
    j. Encourage ventilation of feelings about fear of dying
    k. Administer antibiotics
    l. Administer antidiarrheals
    m. Monitor for infection
    n. Administer mouth and skin care
    o. Assess for bruising and petechiae
4. Possible surgical complications
    a. Marrow graft rejection
    b. Graft versus host disease
    c. Cataracts
    d. Stomatitis
    e. Hemorrhage
5. Patient/family postoperative teaching goals; the patient will:
    a. Keep follow-up appointments
    b. State the action, side effects, and scheduling of medications
    c. Recognize the signs and symptoms of infection and bleeding
    d. Complete daily skin care
    e. Identify changes in vision

I. **Agranulocytosis (granulocytopenia)**
    1. Definition: profound decrease in the number of granulocytes
    2. Possible etiology
        a. Idiopathic
        b. Exposure to chemicals
        c. Drug induced: chloramphenicol (Chloromycetin), chlorpromazine (Thorazine), phenytoin sodium (Dilantin)
        d. Chemotherapy
        e. Radiation
        f. Radioisotopes
        g. Hemodialysis
        h. Viral infection

3. Pathophysiology
   a. Number of granulocytes is reduced because of increased utilization, lack of maturation, or shortened life span
   b. The reduced number of granulocytes diminishes resistance to disease
4. Possible clinical manifestations
   a. Fatigue
   b. Malaise
   c. Elevated temperature
   d. Chills
   e. Sore throat
   f. Multiple infections
   g. Weakness
   h. Dysphagia
   i. Enlarged cervical lymph nodes
   j. Tachycardia
   k. Ulcerations of oral mucosa and throat
5. Possible diagnostic test findings
   a. Hematology: decreased WBC, granulocytes; increased ESR
   b. Bone marrow biopsy: absence of polymorphonuclear leukocytes
   c. Culture and sensitivity: positive identification of organisms
6. Medical management
   a. Diet therapy: high-protein, high-vitamin, high-calorie, bland, soft
   b. I.V. therapy: heparin lock
   c. Position: semi-Fowler
   d. Activity: bed rest, active and passive ROM
   e. Monitoring: VS, UO, I/O
   f. Laboratory studies: WBC, granulocytes, urine and blood for culture and sensitivity
   g. Treatments: saline gargles
   h. Precautions: protective
   i. Transfusion therapy: packed white blood cells (PWBC) and whole blood
   j. Antibiotics: ticarcillan (Ticar), tobramycin (Nebcin)
   k. Antipyretic: acetaminophen (Tylenol)
   l. Sedatives: phenobarbital (Luminal)
   m. Stool softeners: docusate sodium (Colace)
   n. Analgesic: ibuprofen (Motrin)
7. Medical nursing interventions/responsibilities
   a. Maintain diet
   b. Force fluids
   c. Provide pulmonary toilet: TCDB
   d. Assess respiratory status
   e. Maintain semi-Fowler position
   f. Monitor and record: VS, UO, I/O, laboratory studies, stool count
   g. Administer medications

     h. Encourage ventilation of feelings about imposed isolation
     i. Maintain bed rest
     j. Provide treatments: tepid baths and saline gargles
     k. Maintain protective precautions
     l. Administer transfusion therapy
     m. Provide gentle mouth and skin care
     n. Monitor for infection
     o. Avoid rectal temperatures and enemas

8. Patient/family teaching goals; the patient will:
     a. Keep follow-up appointments
     b. State the action, side effects, and scheduling of medications
     c. Recognize the signs and symptoms of infection
     d. Avoid exposure to people with infections
     e. Alternate rest periods with activity
     f. Monitor self for infection
     g. Follow dietary recommendations and restrictions
     h. Complete daily skin and mouth care
     i. Avoid use of over-the-counter medications
     j. Prevent constipation

9. Possible medical complications
     a. Sepsis
     b. Rectal abscess
     c. Pneumonia
     d. Hemorrhagic necrosis of mucous membranes
     e. Parenchymal liver damage

10. Possible surgical interventions: splenectomy (see page 272)

J. Leukemia

1. Definition
     a. Uncontrolled proliferation of WBC precursors that fail to mature
     b. Types: acute myelogenous (AML), chronic lymphocytic (CLL), chronic myelocytic (CML)

2. Possible etiology
     a. Unknown
     b. Genetics
     c. Virus
     d. Exposure to chemicals
     e. Radiation
     f. Altered immune system
     g. Chemotherapy
     h. Polycythemia vera

3. Pathophysiology
     a. Normal hemopoietic cells are replaced by leukemic cells in bone marrow
     b. Immature forms of WBCs circulate in the blood, infiltrating the liver, spleen, and lymph nodes

4. Possible clinical manifestations
   a. Petechiae
   b. Ecchymosis
   c. Frequent infections
   d. Elevated temperature
   e. Enlarged lymph nodes, spleen, and liver
   f. Joint, abdominal, and bone pain
   g. Gingivitis
   h. Night sweats
   i. Stomatitis
   j. Prolonged menses
   k. Hematemesis
   l. Melena
   m. Jaundice
   n. Tachycardia
   o. Hypotension
5. Possible diagnostic test findings
   a. Hematology: decreased Hct, Hgb, RBC, platelets; increased ESR, immature WBC, bleeding time
   b. Bone marrow biopsy: large number of immature leukocytes
6. Medical management
   a. Diet therapy: high-protein, high-vitamin and mineral, high-calorie, low-roughage, bland, soft in small, frequent feedings
   b. I.V. therapy: hydration, heparin lock
   c. Oxygen therapy
   d. Position: semi-Fowler
   e. Activity: bed rest, active and passive ROM, isometric exercises
   f. Monitoring: VS, UO, I/O
   g. Laboratory studies: Hgb, Hct, WBC, platelets, BUN, Cr, surveillance cultures
   h. Nutritional support: IVH
   i. Radiation therapy
   j. Chemotherapy
   k. Treatments: sitz baths, bed cradle, tepid baths
   l. Precautions: protective or laminar air flow room
   m. Transfusion therapy: platelets, packed red blood cells (PRBC), whole blood
   n. Antibiotics: doxorubicin (Adriamycin), plicamycin (Mithramycin)
   o. Antipyretic: acetaminophen (Tylenol)
   p. Stool softeners: docusate sodium (Colace)
   q. Analgesics: ibuprofen (Motrin)
   r. Antigout: allopurinol (Zyloprim)
   s. Tranquilizers: diazepam (Valium)
   t. Systemic alkalinizers: sodium bicarbonate
   u. Antimetabolites: fluorouracil (5-FU), methotrexate (MTX)

     v.   Alkylating agents: busulfan (Myleran), chlorambucil (Leukeran)
    w. Antineoplastics: vinblastine (VLB), vincristine (Oncovin)
     x. Enzymes: L-asparaginase (Elspar)
     y. Estrogens: diethystibestrol (DES)
     z. Progestins: medroxyprogesterone (Provera)

7. Medical nursing interventions/responsibilities
     a. Maintain diet
     b. Force fluids
     c. Administer I.V. fluids
     d. Administer oxygen
     e. Provide pulmonary toilet: TCDB
     f. Assess cardiovascular, neurologic, respiratory, and renal status and fluid balance
     g. Maintain semi-Fowler position
     h. Monitor and record VS, UO, I/O, laboratory studies, daily weights, urine, stool, and emesis for occult blood
     i. Administer IVH
     j. Administer transfusion therapy
     k. Administer medications
     l. Encourage ventilation of feelings about change in body image and fear of dying
    m. Maintain bed rest
     n. Provide treatments: sitz baths, bed cradle, tepid baths
     o. Allay anxiety
     p. Monitor for bleeding and infection
     q. Maintain protective precautions
     r. Provide gentle mouth and skin care
     s. Avoid intramuscular injections, enemas, rectal temperatures, straight razors
     t. Provide postchemotherapeutic care: provide skin, mouth, and perineal care; encourage dietary intake; administer antiemetics and antidiarrheals; monitor for bleeding, infection, and electrolyte imbalance; provide rest periods

8. Patient/family teaching goals; the patient will:
     a. Keep follow-up appointments
     b. Maintain ideal weight
     c. State the action, side effects, and scheduling of medications
     d. Recognize the signs and symptoms of occult blood and infection
     e. Avoid exposure to people with infections
     f. Alternate rest periods with activity
     g. Monitor self for infection
     h. Follow dietary recommendations and restrictions
     i. Seek help from community agencies and resources
     j. Complete daily skin and mouth care
     k. Prevent constipation
     l. Use electric razor

    m. Avoid use of over-the-counter drugs
    n. Monitor stool for occult blood
    o. Increase fluid intake
    p. Demonstrate Hickman catheter care
9. Possible medical complications
    a. Gross systemic hemorrhage
    b. Acute renal failure
    c. Cerebrovascular accident (CVA)
    d. Thrombocytopenia
    e. Perirectal abscess
    f. Gastrointestinal bleeding
    g. Fungal and bacterial infection
    h. Meningitis
10. Possible surgical interventions: bone marrow transplant (see page 273)

K. Lymphomas
1. Definition
    a. Hodgkin's disease: proliferation of malignant Reed-Sternberg cells within lymph nodes
    b. Non-Hodgkin's lymphoma: malignant tumors of lymph nodes and lymphatic tissues that cannot be classified as Hodgkin's disease
    c. Classes of non-Hodgkin's lymphoma: B-lymphocyte malignancies, T-lymphocyte malignancies, and histiocyte malignancies
2. Possible etiology
    a. Unknown
    b. Viral
    c. Genetic (Hodgkin's disease)
    d. Environmental (Hodgkin's disease)
    e. Immunologic
3. Pathophysiology
    a. Reed-Sternberg cells proliferate in a single lymph node and travel contiguously through the lymphathic system to other lymphatic nodes and organs (Hodgkin's disease)
    b. Immune system cell tumors occur throughout lymph nodes and lymphatic organs in unpredictable patterns (non-Hodgkin's lymphoma)
4. Possible clinical manifestations
    a. Enlarged, nontender, firm, and movable lymph nodes in lower cervical regions (Hodgkin's disease)
    b. Recurrent, intermittent fever
    c. Night sweats
    d. Weight loss
    e. Malaise
    f. Lethargy
    g. Severe pruritus
    h. Dyspnea (Hodgkin's disease)
    i. Anorexia

     j. Bone pain (Hodgkin's disease)
     k. Cough
     l. Recurrent infection
     m. Hepatomegaly
     n. Splenomegaly
     o. Dysphagia (Hodgkin's disease)
     p. Edema and cyanosis of face and neck (Hodgkin's disease)
     q. Prominent, painless, generalized lymphadenopathy (non-Hodgkin's lymphoma)

5. Possible diagnostic test findings
     a. Bone marrow aspiration and biopsy: small, diffuse lymphocytic or large, follicular-type cells (non-Hodgkin's lymphoma)
     b. Hematology: decreased Hgb, Hct, platelets (non-Hodgkin's and Hodgkin's); increased ESR (Hodgkin's and non-Hodgkin's lymphoma); increased leukocytes, gammaglobulin (Hodgkin's)
     c. Lymphangiogram: positive lymph node involvement (Hodgkin's disease)
     d. Lymph node biopsy: positive for Reed-Sternberg cells (Hodgkin's disease)
     e. Chest X-ray (CXR): lymphadenopathy (Hodgkin's disease)
     f. Blood chemistry: increased alkaline phosphatase, copper (Hodgkin's disease)
     g. Stage I: asymptomatic: malignant cells found in single lymph node
     h. Stage II: symptomatic; malignant cells found in two or three adjacent lymph nodes on same side of diaphragm
     i. Stage III: symptomatic; malignant cells widely disseminated to lymph nodes on both sides of diaphragm and to organs
     j. Stage IV: symptomatic; malignant cells found in one or more extralymphatic organs or tissues with or without lymphatic involvement

6. Medical management
     a. Diet therapy: high-protein, high-calorie, high-vitamin and mineral, high-iron, high-calcium, bland, soft
     b. I.V. therapy: heparin lock
     c. Oxygen therapy
     d. Position: semi-Fowler
     e. Acitvity: bed rest, active and passive ROM
     f. Monitoring: VS, UO, I/O
     g. Laboratory studies: Hgb, Hct, WBC, platelets
     h. Radiation therapy
     i. Precautions: protective
     j. Transfusion therapy: PRBC
     k. MOPP chemotherapy protocol: mechlorethamine (Mustargen), vincristine (Oncovin), procarbazine (Matulane), prednisone (Hodgkin's disease)
     l. ABVD chemotherapy protocol: doxorubicin (Adriamycin), bleomycin (Blenoxane), vinblastine (VLB), dacarbazine (DTIC) (Hodgkin's disease)
     m. Analgesics: meperidine hydrochloride (Demerol)
     n. Sedatives: phenobarbital (Luminal)
     o. Stool softeners: docusate sodium (Colace)

    p. Antipruritics: diphenhydramine (Benadryl)

    q. CVP chemotherapy protocol: cyclophosphamide (Cytoxan), vincristine (Oncovin), prednisone (non-Hodgkin's lymphoma)

    r. CHOP chemotherapy protocol: cyclophosphamide (Cytoxan), doxorubicin (Adriamycin), vincristine (Oncovin), prednisone (non-Hodgkin's lymphoma)

7. Medical nursing interventions/responsibilities
   a. Maintain diet
   b. Force fluids
   c. Administer I.V. fluids
   d. Administer oxygen
   e. Provide pulmonary toilet: TCDB
   f. Assess respiratory, cardiovascular, and neurologic status and fluid balance
   g. Maintain semi-Fowler position
   h. Monitor and record VS, UO, I/O, laboratory studies, specific gravity
   i. Administer medications
   j. Encourage ventilation of feelings about change in body image and fear of dying
   k. Maintain bed rest
   l. Provide frequent baths with mild soap
   m. Provide mouth and skin care
   n. Administer transfusion therapy
   o. Allay anxiety
   p. Avoid aspirin and straight razors
   q. Provide postchemotherapeutic and/or postradiation nursing care: provide skin, mouth, and perineal care; encourage dietary intake; administer antiemetics and antidiarrheals; monitor for bleeding, infection, and electrolyte imbalance; provide rest periods
   r. Monitor for jaundice and infection
   s. Maintain protective precautions

8. Patient/family teaching goals; the patient will:
   a. Keep follow-up appointments
   b. Maintain regular exercise program
   c. Maintain ideal weight
   d. State the action, side effects, and scheduling of medications
   e. Recognize the signs and symptoms of infection and motor and sensory deficits
   f. Avoid exposure to people with infections
   g. Alternate rest periods with activity
   h. Monitor self for infection
   i. Follow dietary recommendations and restrictions
   j. Promote a safe environment
   k. Complete daily skin and mouth care
   l. Increase fluid intake
   m. Use electric razors

      n. Avoid use of over-the-counter medications

      o. Avoid use of aspirin

  9. Possible medical complications

      a. Metastasis (Hodgkin's disease)

      b. Hypersplenism

      c. Pleural effusion (Hodgkin's disease)

      d. Herpes zoster (Hodgkin's disease)

      e. Depression

      f. Pancytopenia (Hodgkin's disease)

      g. Pneumonitis (Hodgkin's disease)

      h. Paraplegia

      i. Pericarditis (Hodgkin's disease)

      j. Nephritis (Hodgkin's disease)

      k. Hypothyroidism (Hodgkin's disease)

      l. Neuralgia (Hodgkin's disease)

      m. Obstructive jaundice (Hodgkin's disease)

      n. Infections: viral, bacterial, fungal (non-Hodgkin's lymphoma)

      o. Intestinal obstruction (non-Hodgkin's lymphoma)

      p. Leukemia (non-Hodgkin's lymphoma)

      q. Superior vena cava obstruction (non-Hodgkin's lymphoma)

  10. Possible surgical interventions: splenectomy (see page 272)

L. Acquired immune deficiency syndrome (AIDS)

  1. Definition: defect in T-cell mediated immunity that allows the development of fatal opportunistic infections

  2. Possible etiology

      a. Exposure to blood containing human immunodeficiency virus (HIV): transfusions, contaminated needles, handling of blood, in utero

      b. Exposure to semen containing HIV virus: sexual intercourse, handling of semen

  3. Pathophysiology

      a. HIV-infected lymphocytes are carried in semen and blood

      b. Infected lymphocytes in semen are transferred through minute breaks in skin and mucosa

      c. Infected lymphocytes in blood are transferred via transfusion, fetal circulation, and minute breaks in skin and mucosa

      d. HIV virus reproduces within the T-lymphocytes and destroys them

      e. The destruction of the T-lymphocytes diminishes resistance to disease

  4. Possible clinical manifestations

      a. AIDS-related complex (ARC): fatigue, weakness, anorexia, weight loss, recurrent diarrhea, fever, lymphadenopathy, pallor, night sweats, malnutrition

      b. Disorientation and confusion

      c. Dyspnea

      d. Dementia

5. Possible diagnostic test findings
    a. Hematology: decreased WBC, RBC, platelets
    b. Blood chemistry: increased transaminase, alkaline phosphatase, gamma globulin; decreased albumin
    c. Enzyme linked immunosorbent assay (ELISA): positive HIV antibody titer
    d. Western blot: positive
6. Medical management
    a. Diet therapy: high-calorie, high-protein, in small frequent feedings
    b. I.V. therapy: hydration, electrolyte replacement, heparin lock
    c. Oxygen therapy
    d. Position: semi-Fowler
    e. Activity: as tolerated, active and pasive ROM
    f. Monitoring: VS, UO, I/O, neurovital signs
    g. Laboratory studies: WBC, RBC, platelets, albumin
    h. Nutritional support: IVH
    i. Treatments: chest physiotherapy (CPT), postural drainage, incentive spirometry
    j. Precautions: protective; body and fluid
    k. Transfusion therapy: fresh frozen plasma (FFP), platelets, PRBC
    l. Antibiotics: sulfamethoxazole (Gantanol), trimethoprim (Proloprim), pentamidine (Pentam)
    m. Antiviral: azidothymedine (AZT), ribavirin (Virazole)
    n. Plasmapheresis
    o. Interferon
    p. Interleukin II
7. Medical nursing interventions/responsibilities
    a. Maintain diet
    b. Force fluids
    c. Administer I.V. fluids
    d. Administer oxygen
    e. Provide pulmonary toilet: incentive spirometry, TCDB
    f. Assess respiratory and neurologic status and fluid balance
    g. Maintain semi-Fowler position
    h. Monitor and record VS, UO, I/O, laboratory studies, daily weights, specific gravity
    i. Administer IVH
    j. Administer medications
    k. Encourage ventilation of feelings about change in body image, fear of dying, and social isolation
    l. Maintain activity as tolerated
    m. Allay anxiety
    n. Provide rest periods
    o. Provide skin and mouth care

    p. Maintain protective body and fluid precautions
    q. Monitor for opportunistic infections
8. Patient/family teaching goals; the patient will:
    a. Keep follow-up appointments
    b. Stop smoking
    c. Maintain ideal weight
    d. State the action, side effects, and scheduling of medications
    e. Recognize the signs and symptoms of infection
    f. Avoid exposure to people with infections
    g. Alternate rest periods with activity
    h. Monitor self for infection
    i. Follow dietary recommendations and restrictions
    j. Seek help from community agencies and resources
    k. Complete daily skin and foot care
    l. Refrain from donating blood
    m. Avoid alcohol and recreational drugs
    n. Use condoms during sexual intercourse
9. Possible medical complications
    a. *Pneumocystitis carinii* pneumonia
    b. Meningitis
    c. Burkitt's lymphoma
    d. Encephalopathy
    e. Depression
    f. Herpes simplex virus
    g. Cytomegalovirus infection
    h. Epstein-Barr virus
    i. Oral and esophageal candidiasis
    j. Kaposi's sarcoma
    k. Toxoplasmosis
    l. *Mycobacterium avium* intracellular infection
10. Possible surgical interventions: bone marrow transplant (see page 273)

M. Iron deficiency anemia
1. Definition: chronic, slowly progressive decrease in circulating RBCs
2. Possible etiology
    a. Acute and chronic bleeding
    b. Inadequate intake of iron-rich foods
    c. Gastrectomy
    d. Malabsorption syndrome
    e. Vitamin B_6 deficiency
    f. Pregnancy
    g. Menstruation
    h. Alcohol abuse
    i. Drug induced

3. Pathophysiology
    a. Iron deficiency caused by inadequate absorption or excessive loss of iron
    b. Decreased iron affects formation of Hgb and RBCs
    c. Decreased Hgb and RBCs reduce the capacity of the blood to transport oxygen to cells
4. Possible clinical manifestations
    a. Palpitations
    b. Dizziness
    c. Sensitivity to cold
    d. Stomatitis
    e. Dyspnea
    f. Weakness and fatigue
    g. Pale, dry mucous membranes
    h. Papillae atrophy of the tongue
    i. Cheilosis
    j. Pallor
    k. Koilonychia
5. Possible diagnostic test findings
    a. Hematology: decreased Hgb, Hct, iron, ferritin, reticulocytes, red cell indices, transferrin saturation; absent hemosiderin; increased iron-binding capacity
    b. Peripheral blood smear: presence of microcytic and hypochromic RBCs
6. Medical management
    a. Diet therapy: high-iron, high-roughage, high-protein, high-vitamin with increased fluids
    b. Oxygen therapy
    c. Position: semi-Fowler
    d. Activity: bed rest
    e. Monitoring: VS, UO, I/O
    f. Laboratory studies: arterial blood gases (ABGs), Hgb, Hct, iron, iron-binding capacity
    g. Transfusion therapy: PRBC
    h. Hematinics: ferrous sulfate (Feosol), iron dextran (Imferon), iron sorbitex (Jectofer)
    i. Vitamins: pyridoxine hydrochloride (vitamin B_6), ascorbic acid (vitamin C)
7. Medical nursing interventions/responsibilities
    a. Maintain diet with increased fluids
    b. Force fluids
    c. Administer oxygen
    d. Assess cardiovascular and respiratory status
    e. Maintain semi-Fowler position
    f. Monitor and record VS, UO, I/O, laboratory studies
    g. Administer medications

h. Allay anxiety
i. Monitor stool, urine, and emesis for occult blood
j. Provide rest periods
k. Provide mouth, skin, and foot care
l. Protect from falls
m. Keep patient warm
8. Patient/family teaching goals; the patient will:
   a. Keep follow-up appointments
   b. Stop smoking
   c. Maintain ideal weight
   d. State the action, side effects, and scheduling of medications
   e. Recognize the signs and symptoms of bleeding
   f. Avoid exposure to people with infection
   g. Alternate rest periods with activity
   h. Monitor self for infection
   i. Follow dietary recommendations and restrictions
   j. Promote a safe environment
   k. Complete daily skin, mouth, and foot care
   l. Monitor stools for occult blood
   m. Avoid the use of hot pads and hot water bottles
9. Possible medical complications
   a. Plummer-Vinson syndrome
   b. Angina pectoris
   c. Congestive heart failure (CHF)
10. Possible surgical interventions: none

N. Pernicious anemia
1. Definition: chronic, progressive macrocytic anemia caused by a deficiency of intrinsic factor
2. Possible etiology
   a. Deficiency of intrinsic factor
   b. Gastric mucosal atrophy
   c. Genetics
   d. Prolonged iron deficiency
   e. Autoimmune disease
   f. Lack of administration of vitamin B_{12} after small bowel resection or total gastrectomy
   g. Malabsorption
   h. Bacterial or parasitic infections
3. Pathophysiology
   a. Without intrinsic factor, dietary vitamin B_{12} cannot be absorbed by the ileum
   b. Normal DNA synthesis is inhibited, resulting in defective maturation of cells

4. Possible clinical manifestations
   a. Weakness
   b. Pallor
   c. Dyspnea
   d. Palpitations
   e. Fatigue
   f. Sore mouth
   g. Glossitis
   h. Weight loss and anorexia
   i. Dyspepsia
   j. Constipation or diarrhea
   k. Mild jaundice of sclera
   l. Tingling and paresthesia of hands and feet
   m. Paralysis
   n. Depression
   o. Delirium
   p. Gait disturbances
   q. Tachycardia
5. Possible diagnostic test findings
   a. Schilling test: positive
   b. Romberg test: positive
   c. Gastric analysis: hypochlorhydria
   d. Peripheral blood smear: oval, macrocytic, hyperchromic erythrocytes
   e. Bone marrow: increased megaloblasts; few maturing erythrocytes; defective leukocyte maturation
   f. Blood chemistry: increased bilirubin, lactic dehydrogenase (LDH)
   g. Hematology: decreased Hct, Hgb
   h. Upper GI series: atrophy of gastric mucosa
6. Medical management
   a. Diet therapy: high-iron, high-protein, with increased intake of vitamin B_{12}, folic acid, and vitamins; avoid highly seasoned, coarse, or very hot foods
   b. Position: semi-Fowler
   c. Activity: as tolerated
   d. Monitoring: VS, neurovital signs
   e. Laboratory studies: Hgb, Hct, bilirubin
   f. Treatments: bed cradle
   g. Transfusion therapy: PRBC
   h. Hematinics: ferrous sulfate (Feosol), iron dextran (Imferon), iron sorbitex (Jectofer)
   i. Vitamins: pyridoxine hydrochloride (vitamin B_6), ascorbic acid (vitamin C), cyanocobalamin (vitamin B_{12}), folic acid (Folvite)
7. Medical nursing interventions/responsibilities
   a. Maintain diet
   b. Assess neurologic and respiratory status

    c. Maintain semi-Fowler position
    d. Monitor and record VS, laboratory studies, neurovital signs
    e. Administer medications
    f. Allay anxiety
    g. Maintain activity as tolerated
    h. Provide treatments: bed cradle
    i. Monitor stools for amount, consistency, and color
    j. Provide mouth care before and after meals
    k. Use soft toothbrushes
    l. Maintain warm environment
    m. Provide foot and skin care
    n. Prevent falls

8. Patient/family teaching goals; the patient will:
    a. Keep follow-up appointments
    b. Stop smoking —
    c. Maintain ideal weight
    d. State the action, side effects, and scheduling of medications
    e. Recognize the signs and symptoms of skin breakdown
    f. Alternate rest periods with activity
    g. Follow dietary recommendations and restrictions
    h. Promote a safe environment
    i. Complete daily skin, mouth, and foot care
    j. Alter activities of daily living (ADL) to compensate for paresthesia
    k. Comply with lifelong, monthly injections of vitamin B_{12}
    l. Avoid use of heating pads and electric blankets

9. Possible medical complications
    a. Chronic renal failure
    b. Dysrhythmias
    c. Gastric cancer
    d. Gastrointestinal bleeding
    e. CHF
    f. Angina
    g. Neurogenic bladder
    h. CVA

10. Possible surgical interventions: none

O. Aplastic anemia (pancytopenia)

1. Definition: failure of bone marrow to produce adequate amounts of erythrocytes, leukocytes, and platelets
2. Possible etiology
    a. Idiopathic
    b. Exposure to chemicals
    c. Drug induced: chloramphenicol (Chloromycetin), phenylbutazone (Butazolidin), phenytoin sodium (Dilantin)
    d. Chemotherapy

  e. Radiation

  f. Viral hepatitis

 3. Pathophysiology

  a. Bone marrow suppression, destruction, or aplasia results in failure of bone marrow to produce an adequate number of stem cells

  b. Without an adequate number of stem cells, sufficient amounts of erythrocytes, leukocytes, and platelets cannot be produced

  c. Pancytopenia includes leukopenia, thrombocytopenia, and anemia

 4. Possible clinical manifestations

  a. Fatigue

  b. Dyspnea

  c. Multiple infections

  d. Elevated temperature

  e. Headache

  f. Weakness

  g. Anorexia

  h. Gingivitis

  i. Epistaxis

  j. Purpura

  k. Petechiae

  l. Ecchymosis

  m. Pallor

  n. Palpitations

  o. Tachycardia

  p. Tachypnea

  q. Melena

 5. Possible diagnostic test findings

  a. Peripheral blood smear: pancytopenia

  b. Hematology: decreased granulocytes, thrombocytes, RBC

  c. Stool for occult blood: positive

  d. Urine chemistry: hematuria

  e. Bone marrow biopsy: fatty marrow with reduction of stem cells

 6. Medical management

  a. Diet therapy: high-protein, high-calorie, high-vitamin

  b. I.V. therapy: hydration; heparin lock

  c. Oxygen therapy

  d. Position: semi-Fowler

  e. Activity: as tolerated

  f. Monitoring: VS, UO, I/O

  g. Laboratory studies: RBC, WBC, platelets, stools for occult blood

  h. Treatments: tepid sponge baths, cooling blankets

  i. Precautions: protective

  j. Transfusion therapy: platelets, PRBC

  k. Antibiotics: penicillin (Pentids), ticarcillin (Ticar), tobramycin (Nebcin)

  l. Analgesics: ibuprofen (Motrin), acetaminophen (Tylenol)

      m. Antithymocyte globulin (ATG)
      n. Androgenic steroids: fluoxymesterone (Halotestin), oxymetholone (Anadrol)
7. Medical nursing interventions/responsibilities
      a. Maintain diet
      b. Force fluids
      c. Administer I.V. fluids
      d. Administer oxygen
      e. Provide pulmonary toilet: TCDB
      f. Assess cardiovascular and respiratory status and fluid balance
      g. Maintain semi-Fowler position
      h. Monitor and record VS, UO, I/O, laboratory studies, stool, urine, and emesis for occult blood, specific gravity
      i. Administer transfusion therapy
      j. Administer medications
      k. Allay anxiety
      l. Alternate rest periods with activity
      m. Provide treatments: cooling blankets and tepid sponge bath
      n. Maintain protective precautions
      o. Provide mouth care (before and after meals) and skin care
      p. Protect from falls
      q. Avoid intramuscular injections, hard toothbrushes, and straight razors
      r. Monitor for infection, bleeding, and bruising
8. Patient/family teaching goals; the patient will:
      a. Keep follow-up appointments
      b. Stop smoking
      c. Maintain ideal weight
      d. State the action, side effects, and scheduling of medications
      e. Recognize the signs and symptoms of bleeding and infection
      f. Avoid contact sports
      g. Avoid exposure to people with infections
      h. Alternate rest periods with activity
      i. Monitor self for infection
      j. Follow dietary recommendations and restrictions
      k. Promote a safe environment
      l. Complete gentle daily skin and mouth care
      m. Wear medical identification bracelet
      n. Avoid use of over-the-counter medications
      o. Monitor stool for occult blood
      p. Use electric razor
      q. Avoid use of aspirin
9. Possible medical complications
      a. Hemorrhage
      b. Infection
      c. Septicemia

    d. CVA

    e. Gastrointestinal bleeding

10. Possible surgical interventions

    a. Bone marrow transplant (see page 273)

    b. Splenectomy (see page 272)

P. Idiopathic thrombocytopenia purpura (ITP)

1. Definition: increased premature destruction of platelets
2. Possible etiology
   a. Unknown
   b. Autoimmune disease
   c. Viral infection
3. Pathophysiology
   a. Antibody-coated platelets are removed from circulation by reticuloendothelial cells of the spleen and liver
   b. Decreased number of circulating platelets cause bleeding
4. Possible clinical manifestations
   a. Petechiae
   b. Ecchymosis
   c. Epistaxis
   d. Gingivitis
   e. Visual disturbances
   f. Dizziness
   g. Menorrhagia
   h. Hematomas
   i. Increased bleeding after dental extraction
   j. Gastrointestinal bleeding
5. Possible diagnostic test findings
   a. Hematology: decreased Hgb, Hct, platelets; PT, PTT normal; bleeding time prolonged
   b. Urine chemistry: hematuria
   c. Stool specimen: positive for occult blood
   d. Blood chemistry: increased immunoglobins (IgG), complement fixation
   e. Bone marrow biopsy: increased and abnormal megakaryocytes
   f. Rumpel-Leede capillary fragility tourniquet test: positive, with increased capillary fragility
6. Medical management
   a. Diet therapy: soft, bland
   b. I.V. therapy: heparin lock
   c. Activity: bed rest
   d. Monitoring: VS, UO, stool for occult blood
   e. Laboratory studies: Hgb, Hct, platelets
   f. Treatments: daily weights
   g. Precautions: protective
   h. Transfusion therapy: FFP, platelets, PRBC, plasma

      i. Stool softeners: docusate sodium (Colace)

      j. Immunosuppressants: azathioprine (Imuran), cyclophosphamide (Cytoxan), vincristine (Oncovin)

      k. Anabolic steroids: danazol (Cyclomin)

      l. Gamma globulin: IgG

     m. Corticosteroids: prednisone (Deltasone)

7. Medical nursing interventions/responsibilities

      a. Maintain diet

      b. Force fluids

      c. Administer I.V. fluids and transfusion therapy

      d. Assess for bruising, bleeding, and infection

      e. Monitor and record VS, UO, I/O, laboratory studies, daily weights, stool, urine, and emesis for occult blood, neurovital signs, pad count, measure blood loss

      f. Administer medications

      g. Allay anxiety

      h. Provide gentle mouth care

      i. Protect from falls

      j. Avoid intramuscular injections, aspirin, tape, enemas, rectal temperatures, and tourniquets

      k. Use electric razors

      l. Alternate rest periods with activity

     m. Rotate extremities for blood pressure monitoring

8. Patient/family teaching goals; the patient will:

      a. Keep follow-up appointments

      b. State the action, side effects, and scheduling of medications

      c. Recognize the signs and symptoms of bleeding and infection

      d. Avoid contact sports

      e. Avoid exposure to people with infections

      f. Alternate rest periods with activity

      g. Monitor self for infection

      h. Promote a safe environment

      i. Complete daily skin care

      j. Wear medical identification bracelet

      k. Use electric razors and soft toothbrushes

      l. Avoid sneezing, coughing, nose blowing, straining at stool, and heavy lifting

     m. Avoid use of over-the-counter drugs

9. Possible medical complications

      a. Hypersplenism

      b. CVA

      c. Shock

      d. Hemothorax

      e. Death

f. Peripheral paralysis and paresthesia
g. Bleeding into diaphragm
10. Possible surgical interventions: splenectomy (see page 272)

Q. Polycythemia vera

1. Definition: myeloproliferative disorder that results in the increased production of erythrocytes, hemoglobin, myelocytes, and thrombocytes
2. Possible etiology
    a. Unknown
    b. Hypernephroma
    c. Hepatoma
    d. Uterine fibroids
    e. Pheochromocytoma
    f. Lung tumors
    g. Adrenal cancer
    h. Cerebral hemangioblastoma
3. Pathophysiology
    a. Hyperplasia of bone marrow results in increased production of erythrocytes, hemoglobin, granulocytes, and platelets
    b. Overproduction results in increased blood viscosity, increased total blood volume, and severe congestion of all tissues and organs
4. Possible clinical manifestations
    a. Ruddy complexion
    b. Dusky mucosa
    c. Vertigo
    d. Headaches
    e. Dyspnea and orthopnea
    f. Tachycardia
    g. Ecchymosis
    h. Hepatomegaly and splenomegaly
    i. Increased gastric secretions
    j. Weakness and fatigue
    k. Pruritus
    l. Epistaxis
    m. Gastrointestinal bleeding
    n. Angina
5. Possible diagnostic test findings
    a. Blood chemistry: increased uric acid, unconjugated bilirubin, vitamin B_{12}, alkaline phosphatase, serum glutamic-oxalacetic transaminase (SGOT), serum glutamic pyruvic transaminase (SGPT), LDH
    b. Hematology: increased erythrocytes, leukocytes, platelets, Hct, Hgb
    c. Bone marrow biopsy: increased number of immature cell forms, decreased iron in marrow
    d. Urine chemistry: hematuria

      e. Stool specimen: positive for blood
      f. ABGs: normal pO_2

6. Medical management
      a. Diet therapy: soft, low-iron
      b. I.V. therapy: heparin lock
      c. Activity: as tolerated
      d. Monitoring: VS, UO, CVP, I/O, neurovital signs
      e. Laboratory studies: Hgb, Hct, WBC, RBC, platelets, unconjugated bilirubin
      f. Treatments: tepid sponge bath
      g. Analgesics: acetaminophen (Tylenol)
      h. Antacids: magnesium and aluminum hyroxide (Maalox), aluminum hydroxide gel (Alternagel)
      i. Histamine antagonists: cimetidine (Tagamet), ranitidine (Zantac)
      j. Antihistamine: diphenhydramine hydrochloride (Benadryl)
      k. Antigout: colchicine (Colsalide), allopurinal (Zyloprim)
      l. Radioactive phosphorus (P32)
      m. Phlebotomy
      n. Myelosuppressants: busulfan (Myleran), chlorambucil (Leukeran), cyclophosphamide (Cytoxan)

7. Medical nursing interventions/responsibilities
      a. Maintain diet
      b. Force fluids
      c. Assess cardiovascular and respiratory status
      d. Maintain semi-Fowler position
      e. Monitor and record VS, UO, I/O, laboratory studies, CVP, neurovital signs, stool for occult blood
      f. Administer medications
      g. Allay anxiety
      h. Protect from falls
      i. Provide treatments: tepid baths, ROM
      j. Provide postchemotherapeutic and/or postradiation nursing care: provide skin, mouth, and perineal care; encourage dietary intake; administer antiemetics and antidiarrheals; monitor for bleeding, infection, and electrolyte imbalance; provide rest periods

8. Patient/family teaching goals; the patient will:
      a. Keep follow-up appointments
      b. Stop smoking
      c. State the action, side effects, and scheduling of medications
      d. Recognize the signs and symptoms of infection, CHF, thrombophlebitis
      e. Avoid exposure to people with infections
      f. Alternate rest periods with activity
      g. Monitor self for infection
      h. Follow dietary recommendations and restrictions
      i. Promote a safe environment

      j. Complete daily skin care

      k. Avoid hot showers

  9. Possible medical complications

      a. Hypertension

      b. CHF

      c. CVA

      d. Myocardial infarction (MI)

      e. Deep vein thrombosis

      f. Hemorrhage

      g. Peptic ulcer

      h. Gout

      i. Acute leukemia

10. Possible surgical interventions: none

R. Disseminated intravascular coagulation (DIC)

  1. Definition: body's response to injury or disease in which microthrombi obstruct blood supply of organs and hemorrhage occurs throughout the body

  2. Possible etiology

      a. Unknown

      b. Frequent, rapid transfusions

      c. Gram-negative sepsis

      d. Neoplastic disease

      e. Massive burns

      f. Massive trauma

      g. Anaphylaxis

      h. Chronic disease

  3. Pathophysiology

      a. Underlying disease causes release of thromboplastic substances that promote the deposition of fibrin throughout the microcirculation

      b. Red blood cells are trapped in fibrin strands and are hemolyzed

      c. Platelets, prothrombin, and other clotting factors are destroyed, leading to bleeding

      d. Excessive clotting activates the fibrolytic system that inhibits platelet function, causing further bleeding

      e. Acute activation of clotting mechanism results in consumption of plasma-clotting factors that the liver cannot replenish quickly enough

      f. Activation of the thrombin and fibrinolytic system results in simultaneous bleeding and thrombosis

  4. Possible clinical manifestations

      a. Petechiae

      b. Ecchymosis

      c. Prolonged bleeding after venipuncture

      d. Hemorrhage

      e. Oliguria

      f. Anxiety

      g. Restlessness

      h. Purpura
      i. Acrocyanosis
      j. Joint pain
      k. Dyspnea
      l. Hemoptysis
      m. Rales
5. Possible diagnostic test findings
      a. Hematology: decreased platelets, RBC, fibrinogen, factor assay (II, V, VII); increased fibrin split products, thrombin, PT, PTT; positive protamine sulfate test
      b. Urine chemistry: hematuria
      c. ABGs: metabolic acidosis
      d. Ophthalmoscopic exam: retinal hemorrhage
      e. Stool for occult blood: positive
6. Medical management
      a. Diet therapy: withhold food and fluids
      b. I.V. therapy: hydration, electrolyte replacement, heparin lock
      c. Oxygen therapy
      d. Intubation and mechanical ventilation
      e. Gastrointestinal decompression: NG tube
      f. Position: semi-Fowler
      g. Activity: bed rest, active and passive ROM
      h. Monitoring: VS, UO, I/O, EKG, hemodynamic variables
      i. Laboratory studies: PT, PTT, platelets, fibrinogen, fibrin split products
      j. Nutritional support
      k. Treatments: Foley catheter
      l. Transfusion therapy: platelets, PRBC, FFP, whole blood, volume expanders, and cryoprecipitates
      m. Glucocorticoids: prednisone (Deltasone), hydrocortisone (Cortef)
      n. Analgesics: ibuprofen (Motrin), acetaminophen (Tylenol)
      o. Antacids: magnesium and aluminum hydroxide (Maalox), aluminum hydroxide gel (Gelusil)
      p. Stool softeners: docusate sodium (Colace)
      q. Anticoagulants: heparin sodium (Lipo-Hepin)
      r. Hemodialysis
      s. Precautions: seizure
7. Medical nursing interventions/responsibilities
      a. Withhold food and fluids
      b. Administer I.V. fluids
      c. Administer oxygen
      d. Provide pulmonary toilet: suction, TCDB
      e. Assess cardiovascular and respiratory status and fluid balance
      f. Maintain position, patency, low suction of NG tube
      g. Irrigate gently and do not reposition NG tube
      h. Maintain semi-Fowler position

       i. Monitor and record VS, UO, I/O, laboratory studies, hemodynamic variables, neurovital signs, stool for occult blood

       j. Administer IVH

      k. Administer medications

       l. Allay anxiety

     m. Maintain bed rest

      n. Provide gentle mouth and skin care

      o. Avoid intramuscular injections, tape, enemas, rectal temperatures, straight razors

      p. Rotate extremities for blood pressures

      q. Maintain seizure precautions

      r. Administer transfusion therapy

      s. Maintain endotracheal tube to mechanical ventilator

8. Patient/family teaching goals; the patient will:
   a. Keep follow-up appointments
   b. Stop smoking
   c. State the action, side effects, and scheduling of medications
   d. Recognize the signs and symptoms of occult bleeding
   e. Alternate rest periods with activity
   f. Promote a safe environment
   g. Complete gentle daily skin and mouth care
   h. Wear medical identification bracelet
   i. Avoid straining at stool
   j. Avoid use of over-the-counter medications
   k. Monitor stool for occult blood
   l. Use electric razor
   m. Avoid use of aspirin and enemas

9. Possible medical complications
   a. Acute renal failure
   b. Shock
   c. CVA
   d. Convulsions
   e. Hemothorax
   f. Hemorrhage
   g. Coma

10. Possible surgical interventions: none

S. Multiple myeloma

1. Definition: abnormal proliferation of plasma cells in the bone marrow
2. Possible etiology
   a. Unknown
   b. Genetic
   c. Environmental
3. Pathophysiology
   a. Single tumor in bone marrow disseminates into lymph nodes, liver, spleen, kidneys, and bone

   b. Plasma cell tumors produce abnormal amounts of immunoglobulins
   c. Tumor cells trigger osteoblastic activity, leading to bone destruction throughout the body
4. Possible clinical manifestations
   a. Headaches
   b. Constant, severe bone pain
   c. Pathologic fractures
   d. Skeletal deformities of sternum and ribs
   e. Renal calculi
   f. Multiple infections
   g. Hepatomegaly
   h. Splenomegaly
   i. Loss of height
   j. Hemorrhage
5. Possible diagnostic test findings
   a. X-ray: diffuse, round, "punched out" bone lesions; osteoporosis, osteolytic lesions of the skull, widespread demineralization
   b. Bone scan: increased uptake
   c. Bone marrow biopsy: increased number of immature plasma cells
   d. Hematology: decreased Hct, WBC, platelets; increased ESR
   e. Blood chemistry: increased calcium, uric acid, BUN, Cr, globulins, protein; decreased albumin-globulin (A-G) ratio
   f. Urine chemistry: increased calcium, uric acid
   g. Immunoelectrophoresis: monoclonal spike
   h. Bence-Jones protein assay: positive
6. Medical management
   a. Diet therapy: high-protein, high-carbohydrate, high-vitamin and mineral in small, frequent feedings
   b. I.V. therapy: hydration, electrolyte replacement, heparin lock
   c. Activity: as tolerated
   d. Monitoring: VS, UO, I/O, neurovital signs
   e. Laboratory studies: Hct, calcium, BUN, Cr, uric acid, WBC, protein, platelets, surveillance cultures
   f. Radiation therapy
   g. Chemotherapy
   h. Precautions: seizure
   i. Transfusion therapy: PRBC
   j. Antibiotics: doxorubicin (Adriamycin), plicamycin (Mithramycin)
   k. Antigout: allopurinol (Zyloprim)
   l. Muscle relaxants: diazepam (Valium)
   m. Alkylating agents: melphalan (Alkeran), cyclophosphamide (Cytoxan)
   n. Antineoplastics: vinblastine (VLB), vincristine (Oncovin)
   o. Analgesics: meperidine hydrochloride (Demerol)
   p. Diuretics: furosemide (Lasix)
   q. Glucocorticoids: prednisone (Deltasone)

    r. Antacids: magnesium and aluminum hydroxide (Maalox), aluminum hydroxide gel (Gelusil)

    s. Androgens: fluoxymesterone (Halotestin)

    t. Orthopedic devices: braces, splints, casts

    u. Peritoneal and hemodialysis

    v. Phosphates: K-Phos

7. Medical nursing interventions/responsibilities

    a. Maintain diet

    b. Force fluids

    c. Administer I.V. fluids

    d. Provide pulmonary toilet: TCDB

    e. Assess renal, cardiovascular, and respiratory status and fluid balance

    f. Monitor and record VS, UO, I/O, laboratory studies, specific gravity, daily weight, urine and stool for occult blood, neurovital signs

    g. Administer transfusion therapy

    h. Administer medications

    i. Allay anxiety

    j. Maintain seizure precautions

    k. Provide skin and mouth care

    l. Alternate rest periods with activity

    m. Monitor for infection and bruising

    n. Prevent falls

    o. Provide postchemotherapeutic and/or postradiation nursing care: provide skin, mouth, and perineal care; encourage dietary intake; administer antiemetics and antidiarrheals; monitor for bleeding, infection, and electrolyte imbalance; provide rest periods

    p. Assess bone pain

    q. Move patient gently

    r. Apply and/or maintain orthopedic devices

8. Patient/family teaching goals; the patient will:

    a. Keep follow-up appointments

    b. Maintain regular exercise program

    c. Maintain ideal weight

    d. State the action, side effects, and scheduling of medications

    e. Recognize the signs and symptoms of renal calculi, infection, fractures, and seizures

    f. Avoid lifting

    g. Avoid constipation

    h. Avoid use of over-the-counter medications

    i. Avoid exposure to people with infections

    j. Alternate rest periods with activity

    k. Monitor self for infection

    l. Follow dietary recommendations and restrictions

    m. Promote a safe environment

    n. Complete daily skin and mouth care

    o. Monitor stools for occult blood
    p. Use orthopedic devices
    q. Complete daily muscle-strengthening exercises
9. Possible medical complications
    a. Paraplegia
    b. Acute renal failure
    c. Hemorrhage
    d. Infection
    e. Urolithiasis
    f. Pathologic fractures
    g. Seizures
    h. Gout
10. Possible surgical interventions: none

Points to Remember

Decreased hematocrit and hemoglobin result in altered breathing patterns and impaired gas exchange.

Anemia is a frequent complication of numerous systemic diseases.

Alterations in the lymphatic system decrease the body's defense against bacterial invasion.

Immunosuppression triggered by medications or disease requires diligent nursing evaluation of the patient for infection.

Mouth and skin care for patients with hematolymphatic illness increases patient comfort and decreases the risk of secondary infection.

Glossary

Ecchymosis — area of bruising.

Epistaxis — bleeding from the nose.

Lymphadenopathy — enlargement of the lymph nodes.

Night sweats — profuse sweating during sleep.

Petechiae — multiple, small, hemorrhagic areas on the skin.

Index

Notes

Notes

Notes

Notes

Notes

Notes

Notes

Notes

Notes

Notes

Notes

Notes

Notes

Notes

Notes

Notes